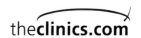

ORAL AND MAXILLOFACIAL SURGERY CLINICS
of North America

Practice Management

M. TODD BRANDT, DDS, MD
Guest Editor

RICHARD H. HAUG, DDS
Consulting Editor

February 2008 • Volume 20 • Number 1

SAUNDERS

An Imprint of Elsevier, Inc.
PHILADELPHIA   LONDON   TORONTO   MONTREAL   SYDNEY   TOKYO

W.B. SAUNDERS COMPANY
A Division of Elsevier Inc.

1600 John F. Kennedy Blvd., Suite 1800, Philadelphia, PA 19103-2899

http://www.oralmaxsurgery.theclinics.com

ORAL AND MAXILLOFACIAL SURGERY
CLINICS OF NORTH AMERICA
February 2008
Editor: John Vassallo; j.vassallo@elsevier.com

Volume 20, Number 1
ISSN 1042-3699
ISBN-13: 978-1-4160-5834-2
ISBN-10: 1-4160-5834-6

Copyright © 2008 Elsevier Inc. All rights reserved. No part of this publication may be reproduced or transmitted in any form or by any means, electronic or mechanical, including photocopy, recording, or any information retrieval system, without written permission from the Publisher.

Single photocopies of single articles may be made for personal use as allowed by national copyright laws. Permission of the Publisher and payment of a fee is required for all other photocopying, including multiple or systematic copying, copying for advertising or promotional purposes, resale, and all forms of document delivery. Special rates are available for educational institutions that wish to make photocopies for non-profit educational classroom use. Permissions may be sought directly from Elsevier's Global Rights Department in Oxford, UK: phone 215-239-3804 or +44 (0) 1865 843830, fax +44 (0) 1865 853333, email healthpermissions@elsevier.com. Requests may also be completed online via the Elsevier homepage (http://www.elsevier.com/permissions). In the USA, users may clear permissions and make payments through the Copyright Clearance Center, Inc., 222 Rosewood Drive, Danvers, MA 01923, USA; phone: (978) 750-8400, fax: (978) 750-4744, and in the UK through the Copyright Licensing Agency Rapid Clearance Service (CLARCS), 90 Tottenham Court Road, London W1P 0LP, UK; phone: (+44) 171 436 5931; fax: (+44) 171 436 3986. Others countries may have a local reprographic rights agency for payments.

Reprints. For copies of 100 or more, of articles in this publication, please contact the Commercial Reprints Department, Elsevier Inc., 360 Park Avenue South, New York, New York 10010-1710. Tel. (212) 633-3813; Fax: (212) 462-1935; e-mail: reprints@elsevier.com.

The ideas and opinions expressed in *Oral and Maxillofacial Surgery Clinics of North America* do not necessarily reflect those of the Publisher. The Publisher does not assume any responsibility for any injury and/or damage to persons or property arising out of or related to any use of the material contained in this periodical. The reader is advised to check the appropriate medical literature and the product information currently provided by the manufacturer of each drug to be administered to verify the dosage, the method and duration of administration, or contraindications. It is the responsibility of the treating physician or other health care professional, relying on independent experience and knowledge of the patient, to determine drug dosages and the best treatment for the patient. Mention of any product in this issue should not be construed as endorsement by the contributors, editors, or the Publisher of the product or manufacturers' claims.

Oral and Maxillofacial Surgery Clinics of North America (ISSN 1042-3699) is published quarterly by Elsevier Inc., 360 Park Avenue South, New York, NY 10010-1710. Months of issue are February, May, August, and November. Business and Editorial Offices: 1600 John F. Kennedy Blvd., Suite 1800, Philadelphia, PA 19103-2899. Customer Service Office: 6277 Sea Harbor Drive, Orlando, FL 32887-4800. Periodicals postage paid at New York, NY and additional mailing offices. Subscription prices are $244.00 per year for US individuals, $358.00 per year for US institutions, $113.00 per year for US students and residents, $282.00 per year for Canadian individuals, $418.00 per year for Canadian institutions, $307.00 per year for international individuals, $418.00 per year for international institutions and $144.00 per year for Canadian and foreign students/residents. To receive student/resident rate, orders must be accompanied by name or affiliated institution, date of term, and the *signature* of program/residency coordinator on institution letterhead. Orders will be billed at individual rate until proof of status is received. Foreign air speed delivery is included in all *Clinics* subscription prices. All prices are subject to change without notice. **POSTMASTER:** Send address changes to *Oral and Maxillofacial Surgery Clinics of North America*, Elsevier Periodicals Customer Service, 6277 Sea Harbor Drive, Orlando, FL 32887-4800. **Customer Service: 1-800-654-2452 (US). From outside of the US, call 1-407-345-4000.**

Oral and Maxillofacial Surgery Clinics of North America is covered in *Index Medicus*.

Printed in the United States of America.

PRACTICE MANAGEMENT

CONSULTING EDITOR

RICHARD H. HAUG, DDS, Professor of Oral and Maxillofacial Surgery; and Executive Associate Dean, University of Kentucky College of Dentistry, Lexington, Kentucky

GUEST EDITOR

M. TODD BRANDT, DDS, MD, Service Chief, Oral and Maxillofacial Surgery, Augusta Medical Center; and Private Practice in Oral and Maxillofacial Surgery, Blue Ridge Oral Surgery, Fishersville, Virginia

CONTRIBUTORS

COLIN S. BELL, DDS, MSD, Managing Partner, Oral Surgery Associates of North Texas; and Adjunct Professor, Department of Oral and Maxillofacial Surgery, Baylor College of Dentistry, Texas A&M University System, Dallas, Texas

DAVID A. BITONTI, DMD, CAPT, DC, USN, Director for Surgical Services, National Naval Medical Center; Staff Surgeon, National Capital Consortium, Oral and Maxillofacial Surgery Residency Program; Associate Professor, Naval Postgraduate Dental School, National Naval Medical Center, Bethesda, Maryland; and Adjunct Associate Professor, School of Health Related Professions, The George Washington University School of Medicine, Washington, District of Columbia

CHAD BRANDT, BA, Owner and Consultant, Active Internet Solutions, Chicago, Illinois; Web and Technology Coordinator, National Foundation for Celiac Awareness, Ambler, Pennsylvania; and Graduate Student/MBA Program, The University of Chicago Graduate School of Business, Chicago, Illinois

M. TODD BRANDT, DDS, MD, Service Chief, Oral and Maxillofacial Surgery, Augusta Medical Center; and Private Practice in Oral and Maxillofacial Surgery, Blue Ridge Oral Surgery, Fishersville, Virginia

DAISY CHEMALY, DMD, FRCD(C), Associate in Dentistry, Division of Oral and Maxillofacial Surgery, Faculty of Dentistry, University of Toronto, Toronto, Ontario, Canada

TIRBOD FATTAHI, DDS, MD, FACS, Division of Oral and Maxillofacial Surgery, Department of Surgery, University of Florida Health Science Center, Jacksonville, Florida

RUI FERNANDES, DMD, MD, FACS, Division of Oral and Maxillofacial Surgery, Department of Surgery, University of Florida Health Science Center, Jacksonville, Florida

STEVEN M. HOLMES, DDS, Director and Chairman, Risk Management, OMS National Insurance Company, Rosemont, Illinois; and Private Practice, South Florida OMS, Miami, Florida

W. SCOTT JENKINS, DMD, MD, Private Practice, Jenkins & Morrow Oral and Maxillofacial Surgery, Lexington, Kentucky

PAUL M. LAMBERT, DDS, Chief, Primary Care, VA Medical Center, Dayton; Adjunct Assistant Professor, Ohio State University College of Dentistry, Columbus; and Clinical Associate Professor, Wright State University, Boonshoft School of Medicine, Dayton, Ohio

EUGENE W. LUCIANI, JD, Anderson, Tate & Carr, P.C., Lawrenceville, Georgia

THOMAS S. MACKENZIE, DDS, COL, DC, USA, Commander, Western Regional Dental Command and Fort Lewis DENTAC, Fort Lewis, Washington; and Consultant to The Surgeon General, Oral and Maxillofacial Surgery, US Army Surgeon General, Falls Church, Virginia

STEVEN R. NELSON, DDS, MS, Private Practice, Rocky Mountain Oral and Maxillofacial Surgery, Denver, Colorado

JOE NIAMTU III, DMD, Group Private Practice, Oral/Maxillofacial & Cosmetic Facial Surgery, Richmond, Virginia

STANLEY L. POLLOCK, BS, DMD, MS, PhD, JD, Professional Practice Planners, McKeesport, Pennsylvania

DAVID B. POWERS, DMD, MD, COL, DC, USAF, Program Director, Oral and Maxillofacial Surgery Residency, Wilford Hall USAF Medical Center, Lackland AFB, San Antonio, Texas

MICHAEL A. STEINLE, DMD, CDR, DC, USN, Staff Surgeon, National Capital Consortium, Oral and Maxillofacial Surgery Residency Program; and Head, Oral and Maxillofacial Surgery/Dental Department, National Naval Medical Center, Bethesda, Maryland

REENA M. TALWAR, DDS, PhD, Assistant Professor, Division of Oral and Maxillofacial Surgery, Faculty of Dentistry, University of Toronto, Toronto, Ontario, Canada

KENNETH THOMALLA, CPA, CFP®, CLU, Chief Operating Officer, Treloar and Heisel, Inc., Orland Park, Illinois

DEBRA K. UDEY, Vice President, Risk Management, OMS National Insurance Company, Rosemont, Illinois

JEFFREY E. WHERRY, CFP®, CLU, CHFC, Managing Director, T&H Financial Group, New Castle, Pennsylvania

PRACTICE MANAGEMENT

CONTENTS

Preface ix
M. Todd Brandt

Dedication xi

Transitioning from Residency to Private Practice 1
M. Todd Brandt

A resident in oral and maxillofacial surgery must prepare for the inevitable transition from residency training to practice as a private practitioner, an officer in the military, an academician, or as a fellow in a postresidency training program. Each career path offers distinct challenges and rewards. This article reviews the issues that face a chief resident embarking on a career in private practice in oral and maxillofacial surgery.

Fellowship Training and Academic Careers 11
Tirbod Fattahi and Rui Fernandes

Postresidency fellowship training is available in many subspecialty areas. This article discusses some of the rationales, advantages, and disadvantages in choosing a postresidency fellowship and/or entering a career in academic oral and maxillofacial surgery. It also discusses factors to bear in mind when evaluating fellowships.

Oral and Maxillofacial Surgery Careers in the Military and Department of Veterans Affairs 17
David A. Bitonti, Michael A. Steinle, David B. Powers,
Thomas S. MacKenzie, and Paul M. Lambert

Within the Federal Services, a myriad of career opportunities exist for the oral and maxillofacial surgeon. The Department of Veterans Affairs and the Department of Defense, consisting of the Army, Navy, and Air Force, have the greatest number of positions available. Federal Services careers are also for those oral and maxillofacial surgeons with a calling to serve their country. The personal fulfillment, patient appreciation, and inter- and cross-specialty relationships are unique to this practice setting because it is free of many of the impediments, to these relationships, that exist in private practice. The highlights of a career in each of these Federal Services are described in this article.

How to Plan a Successful Associateship and Practice Transition 27
Stanley L. Pollock

Once doctors decide to plan and form an associateship, the general process of advertising, recruiting, interviewing, and accepting an associate is important. Here we illustrate the process in three phases. We concluded that not only must the doctors be willing to devote a great deal of time and effort to building the practice but even greater time and effort into building and nurturing the associateship.

Common Contractual Concerns for the Oral and Maxillofacial Surgeon 37
Eugene W. Luciani

Whether new to private practice or a seasoned practitioner, an oral and maxillofacial surgeon (OMS) needs to understand how to handle complicated and often stressful negotiations of contracts for which he or she usually is untrained. This article is designed to give a general understanding of certain common contractual language. It is not comprehensive in scope, but it attempts to cover contracts that are most often seen by an OMS in practice. It is a general discussion of common legal concepts that could face an OMS, but it is not, nor is it intended to be, legal advice.

Credentialing and Privileging for the Oral and Maxillofacial Surgeon 47
Steven R. Nelson

Understanding the credentialing and privileging process is important for all practitioners. Whether applying to a medical staff for the first time, participating in the reappointment process, applying for new privileges, or challenging a clinical privilege denial, the practitioner needs to understand the process and know his or her rights. This article should assist the oral and maxillofacial surgeon and the organizations providing credentials and privileges to make the process less difficult and more efficient.

The Modern Oral and Maxillofacial Surgery Office 55
W. Scott Jenkins

The modern OMS office holds unlimited potential for incorporation of many different technologies. The goal, however, should focus on establishing a facility and environment that is inviting to patients and ergonomically designed for safe and efficient care delivery for the surgeon and staff with an overall reduced level of stress. The possibilities in office design and incorporation of emergent technologies, imaging equipment, and media platforms continue to advance, allowing future OMS offices exciting possibilities in day-to-day operation.

Marketing the Oral and Maxillofacial Surgery Practice Through Positive Employee Relations 65
Joe Niamtu

This article is about marketing. Having superlative acumen on employee relations is much more important to all oral and maxillofacial surgeons than "how to take a referring doc to lunch." Keep a copy of this article handy and distribute it to all new employees. Review the hiring and firing tenets and "Rules of the Game" each time you hire a new employee, fire an established one, or face trying times with staff or partners.

Information and Computer Technology in Oral and Maxillofacial Surgery 79
Reena M. Talwar

> The focus of this article is to provide the oral and maxillofacial surgeon with an overview of some of the recent information and computer technologies available in the marketplace as they relate to diagnostic imaging, implantology, orthognathic surgery, and craniofacial surgery. In so doing, the author hopes to highlight the various advantages and disadvantages of each of these technologies, and thus provide the clinician with a wider range armamentarium with which to treat his or her patient successfully and predictably.

Web Marketing for Oral and Maxillofacial Surgeons 91
Chad Brandt

> Whether you intend to attract new customers, keep existing clients, or expand into new areas, marketing will play an important role. Most small businesses have very limited time and resources for marketing, so it is crucial that the investment receives a significant return. Advertising your business via the internet is a great way to stretch marketing dollars and have the information about your doctors, practice, and services available 24 hours a day.

The Successful Oral and Maxillofacial Surgery Practice 101
Colin S. Bell

> Oral and maxillofacial surgery has been and will continue to be one of the premiere health care specialties in the United States. Incomes of oral and maxillofacial surgeons are among the highest of any profession in the country. With efficient scheduling, organized business systems, efficient fee schedules, and appropriate use of consultants, oral and maxillofacial surgery can lead to a lifestyle that is relatively stress free, allows a direct route to financial independence, and provides a great public service.

The Transition from Resident to Private Practice – Important Financial Decisions 109
Jeffrey E. Wherry and Kenneth Thomalla

> A newly graduated resident faces many new challenges in the first year of practice. Foremost among these is how to handle the newfound wealth that typically accompanies the transition from residency to a successful practice. The ramifications of these decisions are not insignificant. This article explains the important financial considerations a new practitioner must face in the transition from resident to private practice.

Risk Management in Oral and Maxillofacial Surgery 119
Steven M. Holmes and Debra K. Udey

> The goal of risk management in the oral and maxillofacial surgery practice is to reduce the risk of care rendered to patients. Of all the elements of risk management, communication and documentation are two of the most important. Ensuring that a patient is truly educated about all facets of procedures to be performed and thoroughly documenting all aspects of the care that is rendered can greatly reduce the risk of claims. Oral and maxillofacial surgeons should practice these principles regularly and not wait for a claim to occur to teach them their benefits.

Index 127

FORTHCOMING ISSUES

May 2008
Orofacial Pain and Dysfunction
Gary D. Klasser, DMD
and Ramesh Balasubramaniam, BDSc, MS,
Guest Editors

August 2008
The Neck
Eric J. Dierks, DMD, MD
and R. Bryan Bell, DDS, MD, *Guest Editors*

November 2008
Head and Neck Manifestations of Systemic Disorders
Sidney L. Bourgeois, Jr, DDS, *Guest Editor*

PREVIOUS ISSUES

November 2007
Topics in Bone and Bone Related Disorders
Mark R. Stevens, DDS, *Guest Editor*

August 2007
Orthognathics
Joseph E. Van Sickels, DDS, *Guest Editor*

May 2007
Treatment of the Female Oral and Maxillofacial Surgery Patient
Leslie R. Halpern, MD, DDS, PhD, MPH
and Meredith August, DMD, MD, *Guest Editors*

THE CLINICS ARE NOW AVAILABLE ONLINE!

Access your subscription at:
http://www.theclinics.com

Preface

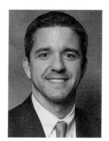

M. Todd Brandt, DDS, MD
Guest Editor

Entrepreneurs and their small enterprises are responsible for almost all the economic growth in the United States.
—Ronald Reagan, 40th United States President, 1981–1989

Management is the efficiency of climbing the ladder of success; leadership determines if the ladder is leaning against the right wall.
—Dr. Stephen R. Covey, Chairman Covey Leadership Center

The evolution of practice management in the constantly changing health care environment poses great challenges to the oral and maxillofacial surgeon. In addition to the basic demands of practicing oral and maxillofacial surgery, issues such as contract negotiations, retirement planning, office payroll, external marketing strategies, third-party payers, and maintaining quality staff can quickly become the focus of everyday practice. Successful practitioners who are also the chief executive officers of their practices understand the importance of efficient leadership and employee management, effectively balancing the complexities of operating a small business while providing quality patient care.

The educational requirements of our profession are as distinct as they are rigorous. Most of us have completed at least 12 years of postsecondary education to become surgeons in our communities. Despite our level of training, many of us have never completed a university business course, much less one tailored to our specialty. Although there may be a minority of surgeons who can rely on undergraduate business school education or an MBA degree, the rest of us sharpen our business acumen through observation, research, anecdotal reports, and the mentorship of our employers and partners.

It is my hope that this issue of the *Oral and Maxillofacial Surgery Clinics of North America* provides you with strategies to enhance your practice, whether you are an established oral and maxillofacial surgeon or a resident planning your transition to private practice. Today's competitive market requires that practitioners be knowledgeable and resourceful to develop a fulfilling and successful practice. Patients are becoming increasingly educated and hold dentists and physicians more accountable for quality of care and patient satisfaction. This accountability applies to surgeons in either the university setting or in private practice. The articles presented in this issue highlight successful business strategies in various aspects of practice management, including the transition from residency to professional practice, associateships, contract law, marketing, and financial planning.

I must acknowledge the leadership and guidance of Dr. Richard H. Haug, Associate Dean for Clinical Affairs and Professor, Oral and Maxillofacial Surgery at the University of Kentucky

College of Dentistry. His forward thinking and selfless dedication to dental students and residents ensures that in dental education, the ladder is leaning against the right wall. I am also indebted to my partners, Dr. Robert M. Driscoll and Dr. William C. Bigelow, who have allowed me to assimilate into their successful practice. Their expertise in business management is second only to their excellent delivery of patient care to residents of the Shenandoah Valley and beyond. Special thanks to an advisor and role model, Dr. Richard M. Nelson, for his professional guidance and dedication to our specialty.

I am grateful to the authors who devoted their time and energy to this issue. Their knowledge and expertise should serve as an outstanding resource for the practicing oral and maxillofacial surgeon for years to come. This issue could not have been possible without John Vassallo, Editor of the *Oral and Maxillofacial Surgery Clinics of North America*, and his capable staff. I also thank my family—Kristen, Spencer, and Cooper—for their love, support, patience, and encouragement.

M. Todd Brandt, DDS, MD
Service Chief, Oral and Maxillofacial Surgery
Augusta Medical Center
78 Medical Center Drive
Fishersville, VA 22939, USA

Private Practice in Oral and Maxillofacial Surgery
Blue Ridge Oral Surgery
54 South Medical Park Drive
Fishersville, VA 22939, USA

E-mail address: drbrandt@blueridgeoralsurgery.com

Dedication

This issue of the *Oral and Maxillofacial Surgery Clinics of North America* is dedicated to the memory of Dr. James H. McLeran, Dean of the University of Iowa College of Dentistry from 1974 to 1995. His guidance and wisdom as a dental educator and oral and maxillofacial surgeon were without parallel. His leadership guided generations, helping to successfully shape dentistry across the country. My career and continual pursuit of excellence as a dentist, physician, and oral and maxillofacial surgeon would not have been possible without his mentorship.

M. Todd Brandt, DDS, MD
Service Chief, Oral and Maxillofacial Surgery
Augusta Medical Center
78 Medical Center Drive
Fishersville, VA 22939, USA

Private Practice in Oral and Maxillofacial Surgery
Blue Ridge Oral Surgery
54 South Medical Park Drive
Fishersville, VA 22939, USA

E-mail address: drbrandt@blueridgeoralsurgery.com

Transitioning from Residency to Private Practice

M. Todd Brandt, DDS, MD[a,b,*]

[a]Oral and Maxillofacial Surgery, Augusta Medical Center, 78 Medical Center Drive, Fishersville, VA 22939-1000, USA
[b]Blue Ridge Oral Surgery, 54 S. Medical Park Drive, Fishersville, VA 29980, USA

As June 30th of the chief residency year slowly begins to glow on the horizon, every resident in oral and maxillofacial surgery (OMS) ponders the most crucial question of his or her professional career, "What do I do now?" For some residents, the question was asked and answered before residency ever began. On completion of residency, many residents intend to practice OMS with a family member or friend already established in the field. For other residents, this question is not answered so easily. Academia, the military, or further training in a fellowship are all equally enticing and rewarding options. This article focuses on issues that will arise during the transition from residency training to professional practice for residents who have decided to begin a challenging and rewarding career in the private practice of OMS.

The beginning

Once you have decided that private practice is the next step after residency, you must face another important question. "Where and when do I start?" can be challenging to determine, and its daunting nature could lead down a slippery slope of procrastination. If you have not done so already, you should start the process now to plan appropriately and leave almost nothing to chance.

If you are only a few months into the first year of a residency, you may think that it is too early to start thinking about life after residency. Although as a first- or second-year resident you do not have much time to do anything other than eat and sleep OMS, you should start asking what you want in postresidency professional and personal life. This and many of the following questions cannot be answered without significant introspection and reflection. You should include your spouse, significant other, or anyone who will be directly affected by the decisions. Remember that you are your own best advocate. If you do not make time to research and determine your goals and options and to plan for the transition, no one else will do it for you.

Each intern or resident should consider the following questions at least 18 months to 2 years before completing residency.

What is the intended scope of your practice?

Private practice affords each oral and maxillofacial surgeon the opportunity to perform every aspect of the specialty in either an office or hospital setting. Under the right circumstances, you can build a facial aesthetic surgical practice, develop a niche in temporomandibular joint surgery, perform the most up-to-date techniques in implant surgery, or administer pediatric general anesthesia. In most communities, however, the oral and maxillofacial surgeon is identified as the dental provider for exodontia, oral pathology, office anesthesia, implant surgery, and orthognathic surgery. Training and state dental and medical regulations determine the procedures oral and maxillofacial surgeons can perform. Although oral and maxillofacial surgeons are acutely aware of their scope of practice, many of future colleagues, neighbors, and friends may not be.

An oral and maxillofacial surgeon who is interested in pursuing a full-scope OMS career must research the area to determine the need for the services he or she would like to provide, the competition among current providers, and

---

* Blue Ridge Oral Surgery, 54 S. Medical Park Drive, Fishersville, VA 29980.
E-mail address: drbrandt@blueridgeoralsurgery.com

the public's perception of oral and maxillofacial surgeons performing certain procedures. Although many successful oral and maxillofacial surgeons provide outstanding surgical care in facial aesthetics, craniofacial surgery, and head and neck oncologic surgery, a large percentage of these surgeons are academicians in large university settings. The reputation you experience as a resident oral and maxillofacial surgeon within a well-established OMS department may be recognized in the surrounding community. Residents entering private practice, however, may find that their new medical and dental colleagues do not have the same understanding of OMS as their former colleagues at the university did. Imagine leaving residency, accustomed to treating panfacial fractures only to be asked by a local emergency room physician on your first night of call if, as an oral and maxillofacial surgeon, you are trained and qualified to treat anything beyond mandible fractures.

A successful transition from residency to private practice requires patience and the desire to educate everyone with whom you come into contact, including referring dentists and staff, hospital administration and staff, and even community members at large. People may ask what you do and follow with, "What does an oral and maxillofacial surgeon actually do?" Take the time to tell them. Be prepared to get some inquisitive looks when you describe the full scope of an oral and maxillofacial surgeon.

It may have taken years for your OMS department to build its reputation and stake its claim within the university hospital and community. You may have to do the same if you are moving to a location where the majority of oral and maxillofacial surgeons perform more traditional services than you plan to practice.

Ask yourself what type of oral and maxillofacial surgeon you want to be and then marry that image with a geographic location that will support your dream. The desire to develop a niche in facial aesthetic surgery as an oral and maxillofacial surgeon is not enough. You must use your own business skills or rely on another's business acumen to find a community and patient population to support such a practice.

What type of practice do you want—solo or group?

Group practice can be a rewarding experience. It offers an oral and maxillofacial surgeon the opportunity to discuss and manage difficult cases with partners who typically share a similar practice philosophy. It can be a challenge as your partners help you grow both professionally and personally. Also, a group practice generally offers a more flexible schedule when planning time off from work, because there are other oral and maxillofacial surgeons to share the daily workload and call. Although group practice has many positive attributes, it can have some disadvantages not usually found in a solo practice. In a group partnership there must be a mutually agreed upon contract for sharing expenses, profits, and losses [1]. You also have to be willing to compromise on some issues when there is a disagreement as to how the practice should be managed. In any partnership business model, you generally will not be able to resolve issues or disagreements your way exclusively.

For that reason many oral and maxillofacial surgeons are in solo practice. If you have a resolute vision for how you want to operate a successful practice and do not want to compromise your plan, solo practice may be the choice for you. It is easy to determine how overhead expenses, profits, and losses are distributed if you are the only oral and maxillofacial surgeon in the practice. Keep in mind that it may be difficult to allot time away from the office for continuing education or vacation, because you will need to have another local oral and maxillofacial surgeon cover for you while you are away. Also, if you were trained to perform orthognathic surgery with two surgeons or if you find you need an extra set of hands during a case, you will need to develop a working relationship with another local oral and maxillofacial surgeon to perform these surgeries successfully. Some insurance companies may not reimburse a second surgeon's fee, so you will have to plan accordingly, determining an arrangement that is mutually equitable.

Where do your family and you want to live?

Where to locate can be can be the most important question to ask before beginning your job search. Practicing as an oral and maxillofacial surgeon in a more rural location or smaller town can be very different from practicing in a larger suburban or urban area. Your scope of practice may be restricted in certain regions of the country, not necessarily by a state's dental practice act but rather by the area's need for your services. Many residents are told to practice where they want to live, whether the area is saturated with oral and maxillofacial surgeons or not. This advice suggests that if you are diligent and a great doctor, you will be successful. Although this assumption holds true for many, other oral and maxillofacial surgeons have struggled in a geographic area because of saturation of oral and maxillofacial surgeons or a lack of need for the type of services he or she planned to provide. Each resident should research more than one locale. Weigh the advantages and disadvantages of each area in terms of practice opportunities and by how suitable the area is for your family. In your research, consider important lifestyle choices including opportunities for spousal employment, educational prospects for children, travel and leisure options, and local cultural features.

Do you want to purchase a practice, work as an associate, or start your own practice?

Most residents begin their professional careers as associates for a solo or group practice for a determined amount of time. Associateships can range from 6 months to several years, with the average duration being 1 to 2 years. At the end of this contract, the associate typically transitions into partnership. Both associateships and partnerships are discussed in greater detail elsewhere in this issue. Generally speaking, an associateship usually guarantees a salary and benefits including malpractice insurance, health insurance, and a stream of patients who were referred to the partners but may be treated by the associate until he or she develops new referral sources. An associate who is an excellent surgeon and works diligently for his or her patients and the practice will generate income for the partners. The practice takes some risk in hiring the associate and also makes a financial investment by paying for the associate's overhead costs—the facility, employees, and equipment required to practice OMS.

Purchasing a practice or building your own practice is an exciting endeavor. Obviously, these alternatives involve increased financial investment and greater risk. Many residents leave training well qualified as surgeons but without the business background to set up a practice from scratch and manage it successfully. Well-chosen business advisors, attorneys, and accountants can make the transition successful for residents choosing this direction. More than one oral and maxillofacial surgeon fresh out of residency has ventured rewardingly into practice as a start-up solo practitioner, learning how to run a small business nearly overnight. Before you plan to open your own office, consider contacting oral and maxillofacial surgeons in another part of the state to serve as mentors or informal advisors. Trying to reinvent the wheel can be costly for a new practitioner, and an experienced oral and maxillofacial surgeon probably would be flattered and able to provide invaluable advice. If you receive a less-than-warm greeting, consider whether your practice will be in competition with the oral and maxillofacial surgeon you have contacted.

How does student debt affect your career plan?

Residents enter practice today with a considerable amount of student debt. According to the American Dental Association, the average dental student graduates owing more than $141,000 [2]. Residents matriculating from dual-degree programs may incur even more debt in paying medical school tuition. Oral and maxillofacial surgeons begin residency knowing that eventually their income will allow them to repay the student loans, but the debt can be a significant financial burden when you are applying for a home mortgage, purchasing an automobile, or financing the purchase of a practice. Consult a financial advisor before the completion of your residency. Focus on the future and what your financial goals are for 5, 10, and 15 years down the road and for retirement. Having control of your finances now will give you greater flexibility when signing an associateship contract and will put you in a better position to finance a buy-in to an established partnership. An associate may not be rehired by a practice on completion of the initial contract. If this contract includes a noncompete clause, the former associate may find him/herself without a regular salary during the time it takes to obtain a suitable position in another city or even another state. Having a savings plan, a "rainy day" account, or a "nest egg" will make such a situation less stressful and more manageable for you and your family.

Do you want to live near a university to pursue teaching in a residency program part-time?

Teaching can be one of the most rewarding aspects of private-practice OMS. Adjunct faculty can add a new dimension to an already successful residency program by bringing additional cases for resident participation. Some oral and maxillofacial surgeons cover the undergraduate dental clinics to teach dentoalveolar surgical skills and medical management of patients in the outpatient surgical setting. Others work directly with residents, covering call and operating cases like any other full-time attending in the program. These oral and maxillofacial surgeons enhance resident education by bridging the gap between private practice and academics. If you are considering this possibility, you certainly should consider practicing in an area that has an OMS residency within a short driving distance. If driving to the university takes an hour or more and/or a great deal of planning, you may find yourself volunteering much less once you become busy in private practice than if the university were closer to your office or home. Having a practice close to a residency program, however, could hinder your ability to treat certain types of surgical cases if you find yourself in direct competition.

Early in residency, consider whether you want to pursue a private practice or military opportunity and possibly obtain a bonus or a stipend for financial assistance during the residency

Residents may be unaware that military programs provide a stipend throughout residency if the individual is willing to commit a certain period of time to practice as an oral and maxillofacial surgeon in the Army, Navy, or Air Force. There are too many types of programs to list here, and their guidelines change each year based on the needs of the armed forces. Contact a local officer recruiter to obtain specific information about these opportunities.

Many OMS residents arrange to have a stipend paid throughout their residency by signing a contract with a group practice, committing themselves to be an associate for the group following residency. This alternative may work well for the resident who knows exactly where he or she wants to practice. Stipends paid over a year or more of residency may be $1000 or more per month. Also, many practices offer bonuses ranging from a few thousand dollars to tens of thousands of dollars upon signing an associateship contract. Although a stipend or bonus can provide tremendous relief to a resident's financial situation, this alternative has potential disadvantages. Signing a contract too early in residency may limit unknown future opportunities. Also consider that even the most successful practice can change dramatically in 3 to 4 years, for the better or for the worse. Residents should seek assistance from oral and maxillofacial surgeons who have experience with this situation and should consider all possible outcomes carefully when negotiating a contract.

The middle

Once you have answered the critical questions that will guide your quest, you can begin a systematic and ultimately successful search for the perfect private practice. The largest obstacle for most OMS residents to overcome in a job search is time management. How many residents do you know who waited too long into their chief year to send out curricula vitae or research career opportunities on the Internet or who signed on as an associate with a large group practice after only one interview and a single tour of the facility? How many of these residents eventually ended that first professional relationship a year or two later to open a solo practice or enter into another, more suitable group practice? To give yourself the best possible chance of finding the most favorable placement for you, begin the job search at least 18 months before your residency completion date.

Keep in mind as you begin this process that you not only have to find the right practice or open your own office; you also have to apply for hospital privileges, obtain a specialty license in some states (which may require case documentation, presentation, or even an oral examination), apply for dental and/or medical licenses, apply to become a provider for various insurance groups, and obtain malpractice insurance. If you are opening your own solo office, there is a great deal more to accomplish, including leasing or purchasing office space or a building, hiring and training staff, and purchasing equipment [3].

A comprehensive timeline can be beneficial in visualizing and accomplishing your transition. Identify every detail you may need to address before your first day of work as an associate or solo practitioner. Give each specific task a deadline and work backward through a calendar to set your goals. Several hours of careful planning over one weekend could save you a lot of headaches during your chief year.

Many residents begin their career search online. The American Association of Oral and Maxillofacial Surgeons (AAOMS) maintains Career Line, a service that allows job candidates and employers to post and search positions and resumes online. This convenient search engine is located on the Association's Website, www.aaoms.org. Instead of sending out resumes hoping that someone is looking for an associate, candidates can save time and effort by using this resource and effort by focusing on opportunities that actually exist.

If a practice is in a growth phase or has a partner considering retirement in a few years, the group may be just beginning to consider hiring an associate. These offices might not have a listing on the Career Line yet, but a resident can and should send out resumes if he or she strongly prefers to live in a specific region or area. A follow-up telephone call 1 to 2 weeks later may reveal that a practice needs a new associate but has not formally begun the hiring process. A senior partner beginning to envision retirement may not have had the time or energy to seek actively for the right candidate. If that surgeon received an outstanding cover letter, resume, and a telephone call, he or she might be willing to bring in an associate a year or two earlier than planned. Remember that you are your best advocate. You should promote yourself confidently and effectively at the appropriate occasion, highlighting your skills, training, and competent, compassionate ability to practice OMS. Also keep in mind that a solo or group practice initially may inform you that they are not looking for an associate, but if they find you are moving to the area regardless of whether you work with them or as a competitor, they may rethink their position.

Never underestimate the power of professional contacts. Many oral and maxillofacial surgeons search for candidates by calling their former chairmen and residency directors. Keep your attendings informed of your professional goals. Your mentors want you to succeed because you are a product of their residency program. Only an academician can understand how truly rewarding it is to see residents lead successful careers throughout the country. Former fellow residents also can a valuable resource. They can give you insight into geographic areas, salaries, contracts, and starting a practice from scratch. Consider carrying a business card, even if your residency does not provide you with one, so that you can make professional contacts at continuing education events and OMS meetings throughout your residency.

During this process, residents should call local dentists in the area of their job search to obtain professional opinions of the practices you are considering. You can avoid unwelcome surprises by talking to dentists and physicians in the area before signing a contract. For a practice to operate efficiently and effectively, the associates and partners involved should be compatible in their personalities and practice philosophies. You do not want to find yourself in the wrong practice, considering what it would take to leave and work around a noncompete clause because of a problem anyone in the local dental community could have warned you about if only you had asked.

After you have researched opportunities and sent out resumes, you eventually will begin interviewing with prospective employers. Most residents have been through enough interviews to handle this step easily. College, dental school, and residency interviews should have made you nearly an expert in this arena. Use the interview to discuss the mission and vision of the practice and its oral and maxillofacial surgeons. You will undoubtedly review each oral and maxillofacial surgeon's scope of practice, treatment philosophy, and the flow of the office. What you might not discuss on the first interview is the overall financial health of the practice. Be patient and realize that if you have planned well, you should have time for a second interview and visit to discuss further the details of a contract, including salary, vacation time, a bonus structure, and the practice's financial records for the past several years. If you are on a tight schedule, traveling a great distance, or will not have time to meet again in person, you may want to broach the subject during the first interview.

Without much additional effort you can add a few special touches during the interview process that will set you apart from most candidates. When you interview for a solo or group private practice, you will meet many people in a short period of time. There will be partners, their spouses, nurses, surgical assistants, front reception staff, and possibly referring dentists. You also may want to meet hospital staff and administrators during an extended trip. As you meet these professionals, write down each of their names when you have an opportunity, possibly at the end of the day. If you cannot remember everyone, before leaving or on the day you return home, contact the Office Administrator and ask for a list of names of the staff and doctors so you can write each of them a thank-you note or letter. Although this task will require a few hours of writing, it is a personal touch that many candidates overlook or find too time consuming. It will set you apart from other contenders and will demonstrate to the OMSs and staff both your attention to detail and consideration of others. Handwritten notes or letters carry more weight than e-mails, so think before sending a thank-you in an e-mail. It is less personal, and the recipient may not appreciate it as much as a brief, nicely worded thank-you on personal stationery. Although writing thank-you notes may be standard practice for some, it is an important detail that many professional applicants today overlook. This small but meaningful extra effort will differentiate you from other candidates by leaving a positive, lasting impression with prospective employers.

After a successful interview you will want to stay in touch with the office administrator and the partners of the practice. An occasional e-mail and telephone call will remind them of your interest. If you are traveling to a continuing education event or the AAOMS annual meeting, let the partners know so that you can meet for lunch or dinner and further discuss job opportunities.

The end

Once your prospective employer offers you the opportunity to become an associate, you will begin the process of negotiating a contract. During this phase you will need the expertise of an attorney who specializes in contracts for dentists and physicians and an accountant familiar with OMS practices. Plan your finances well in advance, because these professional services are expensive. This money is well spent in protecting your interests. Do not review and sign a contract on your own without professional assistance. The group you are joining undoubtedly will have an attorney and accountant involved, protecting the interests of the practice. Well-established oral and maxillofacial surgeons will expect you to do the same. They should not take offense if your attorney wants to change items in the contract. They may not agree to the changes as submitted, but, as the cliché goes, you get what you negotiate, not what you deserve.

Many OMS residents focus on financial remuneration during the first year of associateship. Remember that although the first year is important, the years that follow are far more crucial to your personal, professional, and financial future. You may be willing to accept a lower guaranteed base salary if also offered a potentially more lucrative bonus structure. Loan repayment plans, automobile allowances, health insurance, 401(k) plans, club memberships, malpractice insurance, and an entertaining expense account for referring dentists are all negotiable items. Although some OMS practices may not be willing to include certain terms, it is beneficial to know the range of issues other residents have covered in their associateship contracts.

At the end of your first year as an associate, your performance will be reviewed to see if your collections more than covered the total expense of your contract. Your financial contribution as an associate may even take a back seat to your treatment of patients and your reputation in the dental community. Often it may be easier to negotiate the partnership buy-in if your future partners feel you have become an indispensable part of their practice and the community at large.

Another point to remember when negotiating your contract is the practice's expectation of you as an associate. An inability to meet expectations after demanding a higher salary and more privileges right out of residency may leave you struggling to convince the practice that you are ready for partnership and are a team player. Conversely, the high salary that was offered and accepted may not seem as rewarding once you realize the amount of travel and time required to cover multiple offices and/or call at more than one hospital. Remember that some practices may offer high salaries to attract candidates because of location, workload, or a history of failed associateships. Consider these issues carefully and address them during contract negotiations.

More important than income may be the opportunity to participate in the direction and management of the practice. Being able to attend partnership meetings and make meaningful contributions to the decision-making process is priceless. Although it may be difficult to ascertain if this factor is important to you, be frank in your discussions with the partners if you want to have an active part in the practice's vision and mission. Expressing such interest will reinforce to them that you are not just another employee showing up for work but rather are an integral member of the team.

Once you have finalized the details of your contract and committed yourself to a practice, enjoy your success with your friends and family. You have worked toward this goal for several years and should be proud of such an accomplishment. The next major task for you will be to complete your residency successfully and to move to your new life as an oral and maxillofacial surgeon in private practice.

If you did not negotiate moving expenses with your new employer(s), contact the hospital(s) where you have or will obtain privileges. Ask if they will assist in paying for your move to your new home. There are laws that govern such financial assistance, and most hospitals have at least one administrator who can assist you in this arena. Again, you will never know what type of benefit they may be willing to provide if you do not initiate the request.

By this time, most residents have been working simultaneously on obtaining hospital privileges, professional society memberships, malpractice coverage, membership in the state OMS society and specialty license, anesthesia license, and enrollment as a provider in select insurance plans, if desired. Each of these tasks requires planning and may take several months to complete. Planning ahead will help minimize your stress as you near the completion of your training and will allow a nearly seamless transition to your first day of work in private practice.

A new beginning

The first year as an OMS can be an amazing experience. You will be faced with challenges, both clinically and professionally, as you begin to establish yourself within your community. Although your best referral may be your next patient, you must keep in mind that several factors influence your success in practice. Every new oral and maxillofacial surgeon must work toward keeping his or her employers pleased with his or her performance, providing proper care to patients, developing working relationships with established and new referring dentists, and developing trust and confidence with the staff.

Whether you are joining a group or starting a solo practice, it is imperative that you make time to meet every dentist in the area who may be a potential source of referrals. If you have time, call ahead and schedule a short visit to meet the dentist and his or her staff during a time convenient to their schedule. You may even need to block off time in your appointment schedule for the first month or two of practice to accomplish these visits. Even if you know a dentist currently refers to another oral and maxillofacial surgeon in the area, a time may come when he or she needs another oral and maxillofacial surgeon to see a patient for a variety of reasons. Do not be offended by the dentist who sends you only emergent patients. View each patient as a unique opportunity to provide excellent service and compassionate, personalized care. Also consider the weight and value of the patient's experience. A rare referral from a general dentist can result in a patient so pleased with the experience at your office that he or she insists upon being referred only to you rather than to the oral and maxillofacial surgeon to whom the general dentist usually refers patients. Consistent quality care eventually may increase your referrals from this dentist as well as the "word of mouth" advertising by satisfied patients.

Even with your best efforts, however, some dentists may not refer to you. Group practice can have an advantage over solo practice in that it may be easier to attract a variety of referrals with multiple oral and maxillofacial surgeons in an office who have different personalities, hobbies, and techniques of patient care. If a dentist does not bond with you, he or she may get along very well with another colleague within the group practice.

Marketing, discussed at length elsewhere in this issue, can begin simply by calling your surgery patients each evening after surgery. Briefly check in with family members and answer any questions that may have arisen in the hours after the procedure. A simple extraction may seem routine to most of us, but it may be the first surgery your patient has ever experienced. A 2- to 4-minute call will impress your patients and their families more than any advertisement could.

Another trend in the health care industry is the growing movement for accountability among practitioners [4]. If outcomes of care were based solely on proper treatment of disease, most oral and maxillofacial surgeons would have to look no further than the postoperative visit to ensure the patient is responding adequately to treatment and healing well. All oral and maxillofacial surgeons, however, have some patients who do well with the surgical procedure and respond to recommendations but nonetheless are less than pleased with their overall experience. To limit the number of dissatisfied patients as a new oral and maxillofacial surgeon, you will need to examine patient flow in your office. Patient flow does not refer merely to the architectural design of your building but starts with the referral and first telephone contact with your reception staff and ends with surgery and postoperative visits. New oral and maxillofacial surgeons also must remember that billing and collections and the process by which your office handles payment requests, insurance denials, and overdue accounts are integral in your patients' opinion of their care and your ability as an oral and maxillofacial surgeon.

Thus, the importance of patient satisfaction in the success of an OMS practice cannot be underestimated. Some OMS offices employ patient questionnaires to measure quality of care and, at

> **Box 1. Points to consider during the transition**
>
> Associateship
>   Create timeline
>   Research opportunities
>   Write curriculum vitae
>   Write cover letter
>   Send out letters and curricula vitae
>   Make follow-up telephone calls
>   Schedule initial interviews
>   Send out thank-you notes
>   for interviews
>   Schedule second interviews
>   Obtain associateship proposal
>   Review contract with attorney
>   and accountant
>   Conclude contract negotiations
>   Sign contract
> Licenses
>   Dental
>   Medical (if applicable)
>   State specialty
>   Anesthesia
>   Drug Enforcement Administration
> Professional associations
>   American Association of Oral
>   and Maxillofacial Surgeons
>   American Dental Association
>   American Medical Association
>   (if applicable)
>   Board certification process
>   of the American Board
>   of Oral and Maxillofacial Surgery
>   Other
> Insurance coverage
>   Malpractice
>   Disability income
>   Health
>   Medical
>   Long-term care
>   Workman's compensation
> Patient insurance
>   Enroll as provider (as desired)
> Regulations
>   Health Insurance Portability
>   and Accountability Act
>   National Provider Identification
> Infection control (Occupational Safety
>   and Health Administration)
>   Infection control requirements
>   Job safety and protection
>   Compliance with Occupational Safety
>   and Health Administration
> Hospital
>   Apply for privileges
>   Volunteer for committees
>   Check for proper instruments
>   in operating room supply
>   Review and understand call policy
> Personal finance
>   Taxes
>   Retirement investing
>   401(k) (if applicable)
>   Student loan consolidation

its core, patient satisfaction. Whether you decide to use this technique or rely on informal discussions with patients and referring dentists, you can strive constantly for quality of care and patient satisfaction through a variety of practices.

A patient's overall satisfaction includes treatment outcome, surgical procedure and technique performed, features of the facility, the friendliness, approachability, and knowledge of doctors and staff, insurance issues, and time both at your office and over the course of treatment [5]. Building rapport begins with the patient's first telephone contact with your office. If you want to be successful, each employee, especially those who greet patients on the telephone, must understand the vision and mission statement of your practice. Establishing trust with your patient is crucial and is fostered by listening to your patient's wants and needs. Open communication has long since replaced paternalistic dentistry and medicine in which doctors dictated treatment because he or she "knows what is best for the patient" [6]. Addressing the patient's questions and concerns with promptly returned phone calls and timely communication with referring dentists and medical colleagues also can bolster satisfaction with your practice. If you are joining a group practice, look to the more senior oral and maxillofacial surgeons to learn techniques that have made them successful in the delivery of care and in building and establishing a reputation for high patient satisfaction following treatment.

Summary

Oral and maxillofacial surgery is a challenging and rewarding specialty. Every resident has the skills necessary for success in private practice. If you plan ahead for the transition from residency to private practice, you will eliminate unnecessary stress and surprises as you near the completion of training and in your first few years as a private practitioner. Clearly identify your personal and professional goals before you begin planning your OMS career, and you will always be in control of your future career Box 1.

References

[1] MCGraw SE. What does it mean to be a partner? Practice management notes. A Supplement to the AAOMS Today Newsletter May/June 2005.

[2] American Dental Association. Available at: http://www.ada.org/prof/ed/students/index.asp. Accessed May 25, 2006.

[3] Business start-up and organization. Practice management notes. A Supplement to the AAOMS Today Newsletter Jan/Feb 2004.

[4] Guadagnino C. Role of patient satisfaction. Physician's News Digest Available at: www.physiciansnews.com/cover/1203.html. Accessed May 20, 2006.

[5] Pawar M. Five tips for generating patient satisfaction and compliance. Fam Pract Manag Available at: www.aafp.org/fpm/20050600/44five.html. Accessed May 20, 2006.

[6] Marcinowicz L, Chlabicz S, Grebowski R. Open-ended questions in surveys of patients' satisfaction with family doctors. J Health Serv Res Policy 2007;12(2):86–9.

Fellowship Training and Academic Careers

Tirbod Fattahi, DDS, MD, FACS*, Rui Fernandes, DMD, MD, FACS

Division of Oral and Maxillofacial Surgery, Department of Surgery, University of Florida Health Science Center, 653-1 West 8th Street, Jacksonville, FL 32209, USA

There probably is no more exiting time for an oral and maxillofacial surgery (OMS) resident than June 30th of his or her chief year. Years of hard work have culminated into a finale; now it is time to leave and begin the next phase of one's life. For the overwhelming majority, that means entering a private practice environment as a solo practitioner or as an associate. A select few continue formal training in the form of a fellowship. An even a smaller number enter a career in academic OMS. As the specialty of OMS continues to expand, the ability to practice the "full scope" of OMS is becoming more and more of an expectation for recent graduates. This expectation places increased pressure on the graduating residents and also on the residency programs to meet the demands of the trainees and their eventual employers and partners. In a study on the desired training characteristics of potential associates, McDonald and colleagues [1] found that fellowship training was the third most important factor looked for by the potential employers; fellowship training was outranked only by board certification and 2 years of previous work experience. It is no surprise to anyone involved in the specialty of OMS that currently there is a shortage of faculty and even more so of faculty with expanded skills. The combined expectation for expanded skills and the ability to carry out the full scope of practice has increased the demand for fellowship training.

The expanded training through fellowships fulfills the needs of the community surgeons by providing them with associates who will fill the need in a particular subspecialty and also meets the academic demand for surgeons with added qualifications who will continue to expand the field of OMS.

This article discusses some of rationales, advantages, and disadvantages in choosing a postresidency fellowship and/or entering a career in academic OMS.

Fellowship training in oral and maxillofacial surgery

The American Association of Oral and Maxillofacial Surgeons (AAOMS) currently list several fellowships. Further opportunities in cosmetic surgery exist through the American Academy of Cosmetic Surgery (AACS). These fellowships may be restricted to dual-degree candidates and are numerous in number and scope of training. The training may range from 1 to 2 years and extend from aesthetic facial surgery to full-body surgery.

The subspecialty available areas for fellowship training are many. The following is a list of common subspecialty areas for advanced training:

- Aesthetic surgery
- Cleft/craniofacial surgery
- Head and neck pathology
- Maxillofacial trauma
- Orthognathic surgery
- Reconstruction
- Temporomandibular joint surgery

This list is not all inclusive, but it encompasses most of the available areas for advanced training. The three most commonly chosen fellowships are in facial aesthetic surgery, cleft/craniofacial surgery, and head and neck surgery (ablative and reconstruction). Whatever the particular area of interest, important factors must be taken into

---

* Corresponding author.
 E-mail address: tirbod.fattahi@jax.ufl.edu (T. Fattahi).

1042-3699/08/$ - see front matter © 2008 Elsevier Inc. All rights reserved.
doi:10.1016/j.coms.2007.09.003

consideration when contemplating a postgraduate fellowship.

In a review of factors to consider when contemplating a fellowship, Bernstein [2] stated, "fellowship education has the highest tuition of any schooling you will receive. This cost must be mentioned explicitly, as the tuition is paid only implicitly as an 'opportunity cost,' namely, the money you would have earned by entering practice and foregoing this extra year of training."

Beyond the financial decision, one must choose the area of interest in which to seek further training. The decision is predicated on several factors. The most common reason for further training is to become more proficient in a subspecialty area so that the trainee will have a special set of skills upon completion of the training. The skills gained then will further the individual's career, whether private or academic. Another reason to seek fellowship training is to bolster the skills in an area where training was deficient or in a subspecialty area where the candidate does not feel comfortable performing procedures without supervision.

Once the decision to pursue fellowship training is made, the candidate must decide how to evaluate the existing options and decide which one to apply to.

The following are factors to keep in mind when evaluating fellowships as delineated by Bernstein:

1. Know yourself.
2. Scrutinize the structure of the program.
3. Assess the track record.
4. Glance (quickly) at what you will be paid.
5. Find out if everybody plays nicely.
6. Ask about on-call duties. ("How good?" is more important than "how often?")
7. Look for diversity.
8. Investigate the research program.
9. Don't overpay for a brand name.
10. Give credit for accreditation.

Although the preceding criteria were written for the evaluation of orthopedic surgery fellowships, they apply to OMS fellowships as well. The first factor, knowing yourself, refers both to what it is that one wishes to accomplish during that year and also to evaluating the eventual burden that will be placed on one's family. Although most fellowship offer a stipend, it is very difficult to continue the deferment option on any deferred dental and/or medical school loans. Although the interest on these loans will continue to accrue, most lenders will require some type of repayment once the residency program concludes. This repayment can vary significantly, depending on the amount of the original loan and the lender. Some fellowships, especially facial aesthetic fellowships, require that the fellow purchase malpractice coverage while in the fellowship. This requirement also can increase the overall cost of living. Some fellowships also require obtaining dental and/or medical licensure in that particular state. This undertaking is costly and can be arduous and lengthy as well.

Another important consideration when contemplating a fellowship is the family. Residency can place a significant burden on the spouse and family, as many studies have shown [3,4]. A wise question to ascertain is, "Is my spouse ready for a fellowship?" Relocating to another state for 1 to 2 years and living on a limited income with extended working hours can be difficult on the family and spouse.

The track record is important when evaluating a fellowship. The candidate should inquire about the current positions of previous fellows. This information allows the candidate to know if the skills and contacts gained by doing that particular fellowship are in keeping with what he or she intends to gain.

The majority of OMS fellowships are dependant on the skills of one leading surgeon. In these fellowships the fellow will not benefit from the diversity of thought on management of clinical problems that could be obtained from a fellowship in which there are multiple faculty members with varied backgrounds.

Another factor to consider is the ability to moonlight to supplement one's income during a fellowship. This opportunity is open to any individual who has an active license (usually medical) in a particular state and involves functioning as a physician in an urgent care center, emergency department, or an OMS office for an hourly wage. Although moonlighting can be a significant source of extra income, some fellowship directors do not allow their fellows to moonlight, or, because of the rigors of the fellowship, there simply may not be time available to moonlight.

Most fellowships are advertised on the AAOMS Website, www.aaoms.org. Some also are listed in various journals, such as the *Journal of Oral and Maxillofacial Surgery* and the *American Journal of Cosmetic Surgery*. Although most of these fellowships are within the United States, a handful are available abroad, usually in Europe,

Australia, and Mexico. Fellowship opportunities abroad should be contacted directly because they usually are not advertised as often.

Most individuals interested in pursing a fellowship must apply for a position before the beginning of their final year in residency. Available fellowship positions are limited and therefore are quite competitive. Some fellowships simply require the candidate to complete an application generated by the institution offering the position, but others require supplemental applications through the parent organization (ie, the American Academy of Cosmetic Surgery).

Most fellowship directors encourage the fellow to take the American Board of Oral and Maxillofacial Surgery Written Qualifying Examination (WQE) while in fellowship. Doing so is highly recommended. Both authors successfully completed their WQE while in fellowship and strongly urge others to do so. Completing the WQE in a timely manner allows the applicant to recall as much information gained from residency as possible without a significant lapse in time.

Given the continued expansion of the scope of OMS practice, new fellowships in both existing and new subspecialty areas continue to emerge. The accreditation of the newer fellowships may not be as important to the candidate, because that he or she will be the first to receive training in these areas and will pave the road for those who will follow.

Academic careers in oral and maxillofacial surgery

Academic surgery continues to be the dream of many trainees and the eventual goal of some in private practice contemplating early retirement. The expectation of academic surgery is changing, albeit slowly. Historically, the criterion standard was the surgical "triple threat"—that rare superstar who excelled in clinical, research, and teaching endeavors. Today, such individuals are approaching extinction as the complexities and vicissitudes of all three missions increase [5]. Today's academic surgeon may choose his or her role within the department from several possible areas: as a clinical surgeon, a surgeon educator, a surgeon scientist, or a clinical investigator. This flexibility shifts the onus fulfilling the historical triple treat is shifted from the individual surgeon and is placed instead on the department. The department chair has the responsibility to see that all of these roles are fulfilled with his or her faculty members so that a balance exists between clinical, research and educational activities.

Career goals

The surgical trainee who is contemplating an academic career should have an idea as to the role he or she wishes to fill in the department. Having a clear goal allows the individual to seek appropriate preparation in both residency and fellowship training. Although currently many faculty positions are open at several departments throughout the country, the ability to secure one of those positions in a desired location and department is improved significantly by gaining a niche through fellowship.

Financial compensation

The AAOMS has recognized one of the main detractors from academic surgery, the large disparity in compensation between private and academic practice. An attempt to address this discrepancy, particularly for young surgeons, is the Faculty Education and Development Award. This competitive award seeks to identify young faculty members who have shown a commitment to the specialty and academics. The award supplements the salary of the recipient for a period of 3 years in return for a commitment to remain in academic surgery for a defined period of time. Although this award is welcomed by all of its recipients, the problem of financial disparity still needs to be evaluated and remedied to retain current faculty and to attract future faculty.

Other issues cited as common detractors to the pursuit of an academic career are long working hours, lack of adequate compensation, involvement in complex and perhaps litigious surgical cases, and the unappealing administrative burdens and institutional politics.

Although some of these issues are real, some are not. Many of the best-known OMS surgeons have had very satisfying careers in academic surgery and have fared well in both their scholarly work and in their personal and financial lives. To most individuals attracted to academic OMS, the potential obstacles are overshadowed by advantages such as educating students and future residents, ability to perform complex surgical procedures, and the freedom to practice the entire scope or a select area of OMS. Academic surgeons benefit from certain intangibles: the ability to attend conferences within and outside of the country with fewer worries about maintaining the practice, paid fees to societal memberships, and the provision of office space, support staff, and overhead. Most academic institutions also offer their faculty members attractive retirement and pension plans. Retirement accounts (401(k) and others) can become significant assets because the institution usually matches voluntary contributions to such plans. Also, most of the voluntary contributions are tax deductible. The accrued retirement is transferable from one institution to another.

Recently, medical institutions have placed some emphasis on individual salary lines based on findings of the Medical Group Management Association (MGMA). This group, founded in the 1920s, is the premier organization in the country involved in improving the performance of medical practices and specialty. As such, the MGMA has established various standards and averages for each medical specialty. This value is based on a survey completed by the members of the specific specialty. It is divided further into academic medicine and private practice. When reviewing the MGMA numbers for the OMS specialty, one notices the extremely low number of survey respondents and what seems to be an incredibly high academic OMS salary. Some institutions hold the individual academic OMS responsible for reaching the MGMA targets; others do not place too much value on these targets. The AAOMS has compiled some information on national averages for academic and private-practice OMS productivity.

Conversely, some institutions offer other alternatives to enhance academicians' financial packages. In addition to a base salary, the institution allows a "private practice" environment within the medical center. This practice essentially operates much as a private OMS practice, and its revenues are shared by the medical center and the members of the OMS department as stipulated in the academician's contract. Other institutions offer an incentive-based plan in which production or collection over a set limit results in a large bonus. Again, these items can be structured in a contract. Contracts always should be reviewed by an attorney before becoming finalized. Contracts are open to negotiation. A contract is a mutually agreed upon document between an individual and an institution. Many young academicians entering practice for the first time may not realize this very important fact and simply accept all the terms of a contract without questioning them.

Additional degrees

There has been debate about "discrepancies" in financial compensations between single- and a double-degree academic oral and maxillofacial surgeons. The authors know of no such discrepancy. Most institutions place more emphasis on the individual and his or her level of training than on an additional medical degree in the field of OMS. At the University of Florida Health Science Center, compensation is higher if one has a master's degree in business administration or is fellowship trained. Higher salaries are not offered to individuals who have doctor of medicine, doctor of law, or doctor of philosophy degrees.

Future growth of the specialty

An important factor that continues to encourage surgeons to enter academic practice is the desire to teach their acquired skills to future surgeons and leaders of the specialty. The role of the mentor has been defined in numerous ways. Pellegrini [6] defined a mentor as

> more than a teacher who provides the bits of knowledge to the learner, and much more than a role model, who may simply demonstrate a pattern of desired behavior for the learner. An effective mentor transcends the roles of educator and role-model and serves as the guardian and promoter of the young physician's personal and professional development. A true mentor takes a personal interest in the success of the mentee.

Both of the authors were fortunate to have had superb mentors during their residency and fellowship training, and both are deeply committed to becoming successful mentors and academic surgeons.

The continued growth and vibrancy of the specialty will depend on the ability to attract bright, energetic, and eager residents. Academic surgeons and surgeon in private practice will have to collaborate to find ways to identify residents who have shown an interest and aptitude for teaching and then guide them in becoming the future academic surgeons. The viability of the specialty will rest on how good a job academic surgeons do in providing these individuals with what one of the authors' mentors, Dr. Robert Ord, calls the three pillars of academia: mentorship, surgical workload, and financial compensation (R. Ord, personal communication, 2003).

References

[1] McDonald I, Ziccardi VB, Matheson PB, et al. Desired training characteristics of a potential oral and maxillofacial surgery practice associate: a New Jersey survey response. J Oral Maxillofac Surg 2001;59: 913–8.

[2] Bernstein J. Factors to consider when considering a fellowship. Clin Orthop Relat Res 2006;449:215–7.

[3] Myers MF. Doctors and divorce. Residency and marriage: oil and water? Med Econ 1998;12:152–6.

[4] Rosen D. Conflicts in medical marriages. Ala Med 1995;64:11–9.

[5] Staveley-O'Carroll K, Pan M, Meier A, et al. Developing the young academic surgeon. J Surg Res 2005;128:238–42.

[6] Pellegrini V. Mentoring during residency education. Clin Orthop Relat Res 2006;449:143–8.

Oral and Maxillofacial Surgery Careers in the Military and Department of Veterans Affairs

David A. Bitonti, DMD, CAPT, DC, USN[a,b,c,d,*],
Michael A. Steinle, DMD, CDR, DC, USN[b,e],
David B. Powers, DMD, MD, COL, DC, USAF[f],
Thomas S. MacKenzie, DDS, COL, DC, USA[g],
Paul M. Lambert, DDS[h,i,j]

[a]National Naval Medical Center, Building 10, Room 2103, 8901 Wisconsin Avenue, Bethesda, MD 20889-5600, USA
[b]National Capital Consortium, Oral and Maxillofacial Surgery Residency Program,
4301 Jones Bridge Road, Bethesda, MD 20814, USA
[c]Naval Postgraduate Dental School, National Naval Medical Center, 8901 Wisconsin Avenue,
Bethesda, MD 20889-5602, USA
[d]School of Health Related Professions, The George Washington University School of Medicine, Washington, DC
[e]National Naval Medical Center, Building 9, Room 2529, 8901 Wisconsin Avenue, Bethesda, MD 20889-5600, USA
[f]Oral and Maxillofacial Surgery Residency, Wilford Hall USAF Medical Center, Lackland AFB,
59th Medical Wing, 2200 Bergquist Drive, Suite 1, San Antonio, TX 78236-9908, USA
[g]Western Regional Dental Command and Fort Lewis DENTAC, Oral and Maxillofacial Surgery, Building 9900,
Fort Lewis, WA 98431, USA
[h]Primary Care, VA Medical Center, 4100 West Third Street, Building 11C, Dayton, OH 45428, USA
[i]Ohio State University College of Dentistry, 305 W. 12th Avenue, Columbus, OH 43210, USA
[j]Wright State University, Boonshoft School of Medicine, 3640 Colonel Glenn Highway, Dayton, OH 45435, USA

Department of Veterans Affairs

Paul M. Lambert, DDS

Today, the Department of Veterans Affairs (VA) offers veterans one of the largest, most comprehensive health care systems in the United States, with 157 medical centers or major divisions and almost 900 clinics located nationwide.

VA oral and maxillofacial surgeons (OMSs) enjoy extremely fulfilling careers caring for those who have served in defense of our nation. Currently, personnel returning from Iraq and Afghanistan have challenged VA OMSs with the responsibility for reconstructing and rehabilitating patients suffering from major facial, head, and neck injuries. The magnitude of their oral and maxillofacial injuries provides a challenging scope of surgical practice.

A career as an OMS with VA offers a future that is dynamic, innovative, and collaborative. As valued members of an interdisciplinary health care team, VA OMSs enjoy the flexibility to move within the VA structure and the freedom to practice wherever an opening exists in more than 75 locations in tertiary care medical centers. In return for their commitment to quality health care for our nation's veterans, the VA offers its dentists competitive salaries, first-rate employment

---

The views expressed are those of the authors and not necessarily those of the United States Navy, United States Air Force, United States Army, Department of Defense, Department of Veterans Affairs, or the US Government.
 * Corresponding author. National Naval Medical Center, Building 10, Room 2103, 8901 Wisconsin Avenue, Bethesda, MD 20889-5600.
 E-mail address: david.bitonti@med.navy.mil (D.A. Bitonti).

benefits, educational support, and tuition reimbursement programs.

The hospital-based practice of oral and maxillofacial surgery offers opportunities and challenges that typically are not found in other environments. VA dentists and other dental professionals use the full scope of their skills and knowledge in their daily practice, and are regularly challenged by patients who can be medically, physically, or emotionally compromised. Many VA medical centers offer the opportunity to work in a collaborative fashion with other specialists performing head and neck surgery. Appropriately trained OMSs also independently manage head and neck pathology. All patient care is performed in an environment that adheres to the strictest protocols for infection control and assurances for quality patient treatment.

The VA is committed to a philosophy of technology-driven care that enhances staff performance and improves patient results. VA dentists work with today's state-of-the-art technology that directly pertains to patient treatment. Digital imaging, clinical operating microscopes, dental implantology, cone beam radiographic imaging, stereolithographic modeling, and computer-assisted design/computer-assisted manufacturing (CAD/CAM) are but a few of the advances that are in use by VA dentists, on a daily basis in some centers.

After years of development, the VA now has the most comprehensive electronic health record in the nation. The health record puts each veteran's medical records, laboratory results, radiographs, EKGs, and much more, at the fingertips of dentists and the entire patient care team as they work together to design treatment interventions. The dental record component of the electronic health record is a sophisticated program that allows the clinician to view treatment plans, write notes, and monitor progress while seamlessly recording production data and other administrative tasks. Because the system is linked to every VA facility across the country, the care team can instantaneously pull up a traveling veteran's records to examine critical components (eg, medications, medical problem list, and so forth) while making informed patient care decisions. The VA also uses technology to enhance professional development. Computer-based networking (mail groups), regular teleconferences, and online training enable VA dentists across the country to obtain new information, share research, and exchange best practices.

OMSs with a special interest in clinical research or training find a rich environment at the VA. Many VA OMSs help guide students' fieldwork experiences. Others conduct ongoing research in such wide-ranging areas as laser-guided imaging, chair-side point-of-care diagnosis or disease management using proteomics, and dental implantology. Historically, VA OMSs have been well published in nationally recognized professional journals. These education and research missions are further strengthened by the VA's affiliations with all schools of dentistry and 107 of the 125 schools of medicine. Faculty appointments are encouraged and time is available for active participation. The VA supports 360 postdoctoral training programs, providing a rich educational opportunity that welcomes OMSs as part of the faculty.

The VA Office of Dentistry has recently established a dental practice–based research network known as VA Dentists Engaged in Research (VADER). VADER Study One, "An Assessment of Caries Diagnosis and Treatment," was launched in the second half of 2007. This network is composed of VA dentists who conduct research in their practices to address the issues and challenges that clinicians face daily in treating their patients. All VA dentists are invited to participate. Study areas of particular interest to OMSs are currently being developed, including bisphosphonate-related osteonecrosis of the jaws (BRONJ), hyperbaric oxygen therapy, and earlier diagnosis of oral cancer.

The BRONJ problem is the type of issue suited for investigation by VA dentists and the VADER dental practice–based research network. Although case series manuscripts and treatment guidelines have been published, additional well-designed clinical studies are required.

Those surgeons interested in leadership positions within VA may apply for several excellent leadership development programs offered locally, regionally, and nationally. These include the Leadership Development Institute, Executive Career Field Candidate Development Program, and Leadership VA. OMSs may follow in the footsteps of those who have gone before them, and assume positions at the medical center–level, including chief, dental service; acting chief of staff; associate chief of staff for education; and chief of primary care. At the system-wide level, OMSs have served on work groups dealing with developing clinical pathways for acute and chronic pain management, and diabetes. They have occupied positions at the highest policy-making level, including assistant under secretary for health for dentistry. In that capacity, they have directed the entire scope of dental service delivery, including recommendations for manpower, resource allocation, standards of care, performance measurement, technology, quality improvement, education, postdoctoral training, and a host of other related issues.

VA OMSs may participate in organized dentistry at the local, state, regional, and national level. OMSs may serve on and chair committees and may serve as delegates and officers. Many OMSs have been elected to leadership positions in regional and national health care organizations, including president of the American Association of Oral and Maxillofacial Surgeons.

OMSs interested in a VA career may receive additional information by contacting a medical center in their area directly, by writing to the Department of Veterans Affairs, Placement Service, 1555 Poydras Street, Suite 1971, New Orleans, LA 70112, or by calling 1-800-949-0002. Employment information can also be found on the Internet at www.vacareers.va.gov. Additional information about practicing as a VA dentist can be found at www.va.gov/dental.

United States Army

Thomas S. MacKenzie, DDS, COL, DC, USA

The United States Army (USA) Dental Corps has a long and distinguished history of service to the United States Army. Mention of the need for dental care for the troops dates as far back as the Revolutionary War (1776–1781). It became incumbent on the troops to take care of their own dental needs, often returning to their home to receive the needed care.

During the infancy of the nation, the needs of the soldier were recognized, yet they were not met. During the Mexican War (1846–1848), civilian providers were sought by the soldiers to meet their dental needs. If no providers were available, physicians would attempt to treat them, although it was shown they were ill prepared to provide much help.

As dentistry progressed as a profession, organized dentistry continually advised the military that they needed to take care of the dental heath of their soldiers. During the Civil War, not much changed on the Union side, although on the Confederate side, several dentists were paid to take care of soldiers.

In 1901, the first dentists were employed as contractors and attached to the Medical Corps, marking the beginning of the Army Dental Corps. In 1911, a bill was passed formally establishing the Army Dental Corps.

Graduate dental education was first established in 1921. The need for specialists was becoming apparent and the Army planned to train three dentists in various specialties. In 1931, the first dental officer was sent for specialized training in oral surgery.

Currently, the United States Army has six oral and maxillofacial surgery residency training programs training nine residents per year in a 4-year comprehensive training program. The training sites currently accredited by the American Dental Association are: Walter Reed Army Medical Center, Washington, DC; Eisenhower Army Medical Center, Augusta, GA; Brooke Army Medical Center, San Antonio, TX; Madigan Army Medical Center, Tacoma, WA; Tripler Army Medical Center, Honolulu, HI; and Womack Army Medical Center, Fort Bragg, NC.

The selection process for admission to training in an Army oral and maxillofacial surgery program has changed dramatically over the past several years. In the past, an officer came into the Army and performed duties as a general dentist for a period of time, before being selected for residency training. Usually, an officer would align himself/herself into a position where he/she could show his/her interest and abilities in the surgical arena. It was not uncommon for an aspiring officer to be assigned as the clinic "exodontist," which allowed the officer to become very proficient and efficient in exodontia.

In the 1980s, the Army Dental Corps' strength numbered over 1700 active duty officers. Currently, the corps strength is less than 1000 dental officers in the ranks. This decrease has had an effect on the applicant pool applying for residency and, consequently, the number of qualified applicants has decreased. The policy in the 1980s did not allow an officer to apply for specialty training until he/she had completed 4 years of active duty in the dental corps. As the number of available applicants declined, the policy began to change to allow younger officers to apply. Currently, an applicant who is on a health professional scholarship program can apply for an Army residency and begin training directly out of dental school, which is similar to the civilian training model.

To be considered, an applicant must submit an application, transcripts from his/her dental school, and national board scores. The applicant must also obtain letters of recommendation, including one letter from an Army OMS. Also available to the officer is a 1-week visit to an Army oral and maxillofacial surgery residency program, during which time the candidate is able to shadow the residents. This visit gives the candidate an opportunity to experience the resident's lifestyle before committing to a residency.

The United States Army Dental Corps selects applicants for residency training once a year. A board is convened in Washington, DC, to select candidates for all residency training programs sponsored by the Army. The board consists of a member of each specialty, along with a unit commander. Each applicant is independently rated by each board member and is then ranked by an Order of Merit list. The applicants are said to be fully qualified or not qualified and are then selected for each specialty program, based on this Order of Merit list and the number of available positions. The recommendation of the board goes to the chief of the Army Dental Corps for approval.

Once the list is approved, Human Resources Command, in consultation with the consultant to the surgeon general in each specialty, assigns residents to the locations for their training. The assignments are based on the Order of Merit list and the applicant's desires.

Oral and maxillofacial surgery residency training in the Army is similar to training in a civilian program. All the training programs are now 4-year certificate programs. Residents spend time in the hospital setting and in the clinical oral and maxillofacial surgery setting. All aspects of oral and maxillofacial surgery training are conducted as a part of the residency, and include pediatrics, adult care, and geriatrics. Comprehensive anesthesia training is accomplished in the main operating room and on weekly ambulatory general anesthesia days held in the clinic. Army oral and maxillofacial surgery residents are well trained in "intubated" anesthesia.

One of the mainstays of Army training programs has always been orthognathic surgery. Because of the economics of a military program, these cases have few constraints. The residents gain experience in pathology, dental implants, cosmetic surgery, exodontia, and trauma treatment, and see pediatric and geriatric patients.

After residency, most new surgeons are assigned to a utilization tour. Each Army base worldwide has at least one OMS assigned to it or one in the immediate vicinity for referral of patients. The new surgeon hones his/her skills during this 3- to 4-year assignment and works to become board certified by the American Board of Oral and Maxillofacial Surgery.

Army OMSs are an integral part of the wartime trauma team. Each combat support hospital has an assigned OMS. The surgeons are assigned to a combat support hospital in a war zone for 6-month periods of time. They are heavily involved in the stabilization of maxillofacial injuries for transport to a tertiary care facility. Most trauma patients are moved to Germany and then to a medical center in the continental United States for definitive care. A patient can be in the war zone and then back stateside within 48 hours. Many advances in maxillofacial trauma care have come from the Army OMS on the battlefield.

Army OMSs can progress in their careers to an academic environment and a clinical environment. As they progress in rank and experience, they can join a residency program as a staff surgeon and progress to becoming a program director in one of the six residency training programs administered by the Army.

Another avenue for an OMS to pursue is to become a commander of a dental unit, either a field unit or a garrison unit. Once in the command structure, he/she could progress all the way to becoming the chief of the Army Dental Corps, a major general flag officer position.

Annual pay is based on rank, number of years in the military, board certification, and specialty. OMSs are the highest paid dental professional in the Army. All service members receive a monthly housing allowance. Other benefits of military service are 30 days of paid vacation each year; paid holidays; a 20-year retirement; free health care for the service member and his/her family; free dental care for the service member and an affordable dental insurance plan for family members; and increased purchasing power in the post exchange (department store) and commissary (grocery store).

United States Navy

Michael A. Steinle, DMD, CDR, DC, USN

The United States Navy (USN) Dental Corps has a long and storied history in the United States Navy, of which OMSs have played an important role. Although officially established nearly 100 years ago, on 22 August 1922, the dawn of Navy dentistry can really be traced back to April 1873, when Thomas O. Walton of Annapolis, MD, was the first dentist appointed to serve as an officer in the Navy. Prior to the commissioning of Dr. Walton, the dental needs of sailors were initially assigned either to civilian dentists ashore or to Medical Corps officers onboard ships; shortly thereafter, hospital corpsmen, with little experience in dentistry, were given the responsibility. The treatment that could be given was meager and thus the need for dentists like Dr. Walton was recognized.

To rectify the situation, the Bureau of Medicine and Surgery drafted a Navy Dental Bill to authorize the employment of civilian dentists at large Navy facilities in the United States and abroad. Even as the text of this bill evolved to the appointment of dental surgeons to military rank, the Dental Bill was rejected year after year by Congress. In August 1912, during the presidency of William H. Taft, a man with a passion for sweets, Congress passed the act that established the Navy Dental Corps.

The Secretary of the Navy was now authorized to appoint no more than 30 acting assistant dental surgeons to be a part of the Medical Department. In October 1912, Emory Bryant and William Cogan became the first two dental officers to enter active duty with the Navy. Just over 1 year later, the Surgeon General reported to the Secretary of the Navy that the Medical Department now had the ability to provide dental care that would allow the Navy to accept recruits who would otherwise be rejected for defective teeth.

When the United States entered World War I on 6 April 1917, 35 dental officers were on active duty, a number that grew to 500 by the war's end. Most of the regular officers commissioned during the war were assigned to ships or overseas activities. Thirty dental officers served with the US Marines in France. Two achieved the exceptional distinction of being awarded the Medal of Honor. Lieutenant Junior Grade Alexander G. Lyle received the Medal of Honor while serving with the 5th Regiment, US Marines. Lieutenant Junior Grade Weeden E. Osborne, the first Navy officer to meet death fighting overseas in the war, was awarded the Medal of Honor for heroism while serving with the 6th Regiment, US Marines.

The war established the general recognition of the value of dentistry in the Navy. Early in 1922, two significant milestones occurred: the establishment of the US Naval Dental School and the creation of a dental division in the Bureau of Medicine and Surgery. By 1941, 759 dental officers were on active duty at 347 dental facilities. Two Dental Corps officers were killed in the attack on Pearl Harbor, Lieutenant Commander Hugh R. Alexander, aboard USS *Oklahoma* (BB-37) and Lieutenant Commander Thomas E. Crowley, aboard USS *Arizona* (BB-39). Less than a month later, the Surgeon General directed that all dental officers become proficient in the treatment of casualties, so that, in addition to performing their regular duties, they could assist in sick bays and operating rooms, administer supportive therapy, and give anesthetics. Dental officers, assisted by dental technicians, performed such duties heroically and, in some instances, at the cost of their own lives.

Revolutionizing the field of dentistry worldwide, researchers at the Naval Dental School developed pioneer models of the dental air turbine hand piece and ultrasonic vibrating instruments. These concepts were a tremendous leap forward for the dental profession. Today, these prototypes are displayed at the Smithsonian Institution in Washington, DC. In 1975, the nuclear-powered aircraft carrier, USS *Nimitz* (CVN-68) was commissioned with the most modern and capable dental facility afloat, supporting seven dental operating rooms, a prosthetic laboratory, central sterilization room, x-ray suite, and preventive dentistry room. When a Navy jet crashed on *Nimitz*'s flight deck on 26 May 1981, killing 14 and injuring 48, dental personnel were integral to the mass casualty response and the overall team effort by the medical and dental departments.

The tragic bombing of Marine Headquarters and Barracks of Battalion Landing Team 1/8 of the 24th Marine Amphibious Unit at the Beirut International Airport in 1983 left 241 American servicemen dead. The only on-scene Navy physician was killed, along with 18 hospital corpsmen. Two dental officers, assigned to the 24th Marine Amphibious Unit, coordinated emergency trauma care with 15 hospital corpsmen and treated 65 casualties in the first 2 hours after the explosion. Both were later awarded Bronze Stars for their leadership and emergency medical services.

In July 1984, the Navy began conversion of two supertankers to hospital ships. USNS *Mercy* (T-AH 19) and USNS *Comfort* (T-AH 20) were placed in service in December 1986 and August 1987, respectively. With 1000 beds and 12 operating rooms, each ship can provide comprehensive oral and maxillofacial surgical services, in addition to those services normally provided by a modern 1000-bed hospital. With the Iraqi invasion of Kuwait in August 1990, and the Operation Iraqi Freedom campaign to remove the Iraqi regime from power, the hospital ships *Comfort* and *Mercy* brought their assets to the war effort. The Navy Dental Corps celebrates 95 years of tradition, progress, and opportunity while responding to the exponentially increasing challenges of the 21st century.

Throughout the history of the United States Navy Dental Corps, OMSs have played a vital role. Currently, OMSs fill a wide array of positions across the globe. As with all specialties, residency training lays the foundation. The selection process begins early, 16 months before initiation of training. Beginning with third-year dental students enrolled in various Navy scholarship programs and extending to senior dental officers, applications come from a wide variety of candidates. Applications are evaluated on several criteria, including undergraduate and graduate grade point average, class standing, letters of evaluation, and National Board scores. Beyond that, candidates are evaluated for military service, professionalism, work ethic, conduct, and military bearing, which provides for a diverse background, with many candidates possessing various clinical and leadership experiences. With training programs at the Naval Medical Center San Diego, the Naval Medical Center Portsmouth, and the National Naval Medical Center Bethesda, six residents are enrolled annually in a 4-year certificate program. Additionally, many qualified applicants are sent to an array of civilian residencies as Navy-sponsored residents. This outstanding opportunity allows residents to attend a civilian residency program while being paid the salary of a Naval Officer.

Each of the Navy residency programs brings an educational opportunity comparable to any civilian program. A full, broad scope of practice gives residents significant hands-on experience in orthognathic surgery, cosmetic surgery, endosseous implants, pathology, trauma, dentoalveolar surgery, and temporomandibular joint procedures. Each program is staffed with four full-time board-certified OMSs and a prosthodontist, pediatric dentist, orthodontist, and orofacial pain specialist, in addition to a comprehensively trained general dentist. General practice residency programs are also affiliated with each of the residencies. Over the past 10 years, every OMS who graduated from a Navy in-service program has become board certified. The Navy also sponsors OMSs for fellowship training opportunities in cosmetic and reconstructive surgery. OMSs can also join the Navy by way of general direct accession and are eligible for the same advanced fellowship training opportunities as active-duty trained personnel. The financial assistance program is another program for non–active duty residents who are interested in a career in the Navy as an OMS on graduation from their residencies. This program provides a bonus, a stipend, and money toward tuition, fees, and equipment.

After completion of training, a new world of opportunities arises. From hospitals to clinics, sea to shore, overseas to the continental United States, the Navy OMS selects his/her career path. Working closely with the Oral and Maxillofacial Surgery Specialty Advisor to the Surgeon General, each billet (job position) is filled. More than 80 billets are dedicated to OMSs, which does not include other opportunities to enhance a military or professional career. Navy OMSs practice in state-of-the-art facilities with the opportunity to use the latest technology in support of their practice. Digital radiography and cone-beam CT imaging, along with lasers and piezoelectric equipment, are available at many facilities. In addition, stereolithographic modeling, computer-assisted treatment planning software, hyperbaric oxygen therapy, and implant planning software are available and used to facilitate and enhance the treatment of patients with extensive maxillofacial trauma, tumor and reconstructive surgical needs, and craniofacial anomalies.

Currently, OMSs have leadership roles throughout Navy Medicine, including Residency Directors, Clinic Directors, Director for Surgical Service, Director of Dental Service, Executive Officer (civilian equivalent of Vice President of a hospital), Commanding Officer (civilian equivalent to the Chief Executive Officer of a hospital), the Deputy to the Chief of the Navy Dental Corps, and the Assistant to the Deputy Surgeon General. As rank and experience increase, exposure to these opportunities becomes available. The interested OMS can tailor his/her career to his/her areas of interest, be they clinical, administrative, research, education, or a combination of each, as the officer desires. The group practice setting of the military is unique and the camaraderie of consulting fellow specialists or members of other specialties for the optimum treatment of one's patient is one of the best benefits of service as a Navy OMS.

As evident from the history of the United States Navy Dental Corps, Navy Medicine provides care for Sailors and Marines alike. Each of the nuclear-powered aircraft carriers requires that an OMS be assigned as a part of the ship's company. Besides providing routine surgical care in an office-based setting, the ship's OMS supplements the anesthesia provider and the general surgeon in times of emergency. A well-equipped operating room can support nearly any maxillofacial requirement. Similarly, when the Marines deploy, Navy medicine joins to support the mission. Currently, Navy oral and maxillofacial surgery supplies one provider in support of Operation Iraqi Freedom. On a 6-month rotation cycle in Kuwait, this surgeon provides immediate stabilization in-theater until transport can be provided for definitive care at a tertiary facility like the National Naval Medical Center Bethesda or the Naval Medical Center San Diego.

Besides the operational commitments of ships and the Marines, Navy OMSs provide various shore-based care. Overseas billets, such as those in Rota (Spain), Naples (Italy), Guam, and Okinawa and Sasebo (Japan), all serve to provide excellent care to the active-duty members stationed at those facilities and their families. Through clinical procedures and community hospital settings, Navy OMSs refine their skills, similar to any civilian practitioner. Having gained leadership experience, careers can progress in various directions, including clinic directors, residency program directors, and hospital department chairmen. Each provides outstanding experience, which is easily transferred to a position in the civilian sector.

OMSs interested in a Navy career may receive additional information by contacting their local Navy medical recruiter; by writing to the Navy Dental Corps, Career Planner, Bureau of Medicine and Surgery, 2300 E Street NW, Washington, DC 20372-5300; or by calling 202-762-3407. Employment information can also be found on the Internet at www.navy.com/careers. Additional information about practicing as a Navy dentist can be found at www.navy.com.

United States Air Force

David B. Powers, DMD, MD, COL DC, USAF

The United States Air Force (USAF) Dental Corps was established in 1949 with the creation of the Air Force Medical Service. The oral and maxillofacial surgery residency program at Wilford Hall USAF Medical Center on Lackland Air Force Base (AFB) in San Antonio, Texas, was the first dental residency in the USAF Dental Corps and graduated its first residents in 1959. An additional oral and maxillofacial surgery residency training program, at David Grant USAF Medical Center on Travis AFB in Fairfield, California, was conceived 10 years later and graduated the first of its residents in 1971.

In addition to graduation from either of the two Air Force in-service oral and maxillofacial surgery residencies, opportunities exist to become an OMS in the USAF Dental Corps by being selected for Air Force–sponsored training at an accredited civilian oral and maxillofacial surgery training program or by general accession directly into the Air Force as an OMS. Financial assistance programs do exist through the USAF recruiting services for oral and maxillofacial surgery residents in training who are interested in joining the USAF Dental Corps on graduation from their residencies.

Since 1996, of the 69 individuals who have begun their careers as OMSs in the USAF, 81% were trained within one of the two Air Force programs, 7% received their training by way of Air Force sponsorship at a civilian program, and 12% entered as general accessions to the USAF Dental Corps.

A wide range of career opportunities exists for the OMS within the Air Force. The USAF Dental Corps has well established career opportunities, or career vectors, in clinical, educational, and leadership roles that are available to all Air Force dental officers. The vast majority of Air Force OMSs are involved in all three career vectors, in various proportions, depending on their respective levels of experience, interests, and aptitudes. Additionally, the size and particular mission of individual duty assignments and locations often influences the role of the OMS at that particular base.

The more junior-grade Air Force OMSs (captains and majors) usually begin their careers with a significant emphasis on their roles as clinicians. Depending on the location, they may also become involved in the academic career vector as a junior faculty member for one of the Air Force's many advanced education in general dentistry (AEGD) programs. In general, as OMSs' experience and time in the Air Force increases, opportunities to assume a larger role in postgraduate dental education and in the administration of clinical operations, or leadership career vector, become available.

The more senior-grade Air Force OMSs (lieutenant colonels and colonels) continue in their clinical capacities but have an even greater opportunity to become involved in graduate dental education, both in the AEGD and in oral and maxillofacial surgery residency programs, and in the leadership career vector in various administrative and command roles. Senior OMSs at any duty location function as the Department Chief in their capacity as Element or Flight Commander. Their responsibilities include overseeing the daily operations and administration of the oral and maxillofacial surgery department and the personnel, both officer and enlisted, assigned therein. Element or flight commanders still have a significant clinical role and are likely to be key senior faculty members within the associated AEGD programs.

In Air Force parlance, the next organizational level above Flight Commander is that of Squadron Commander. The squadron commander oversees the operations and administration of the entire department of dentistry and all the dental officers and technicians assigned therein. Senior dental officers, including OMSs, are eligible to request assignment to squadron command positions, and are encouraged to do so, as their careers within the USAF Dental Corps progress. In this capacity, they still maintain some clinical and educational duties but their command and administrative responsibilities increase proportionately.

The next level of leadership is that of Group Commander. Opportunities also exist in this realm for any Air Force dental officer who has demonstrated the requisite interest, aptitude, and leadership potential to manage much larger organizations, beyond that of just dental personnel and operations, within the Air Force Medical Service.

As stated, multiple opportunities exist for the Air Force OMS to become involved in education. Thirteen of the 14 stateside locations to which Air Force OMSs are assigned maintain AEGD programs. Additionally, a total of 11 full-time faculty positions are available within the Air Force oral and maxillofacial surgery residency programs at Wilford Hall and David Grant Medical Centers. Included therein are two program chairmen and two residency program director positions. These individuals function identically to their civilian counterparts and are responsible for the daily operations, educational curriculum, and accreditation of the Air Force's two oral and maxillofacial surgery residency training programs.

Currently, a total of 22 duty assignment locations worldwide have at least one Air Force OMS assigned to them. Among those, and excluding the oral and maxillofacial surgery training programs at Travis AFB and Lackland AFB, 13 have two assigned OMSs, and the remaining 7 have one.

As mentioned, 14 duty assignment locations within the continental United States are being manned by Air Force OMSs and all but one of those locations maintains an AEGD program. Several are located in or near some of the larger metropolitan centers in the United States, such as Washington, DC, San Francisco, Las Vegas, San Antonio, Saint Louis, and Omaha. Locations where Air Force OMSs are currently stationed include Anchorage (Alaska), Japan, and the Republic of Korea in the Pacific Command, and the United Kingdom and Germany in the European Command.

Air Force OMSs enjoy a full-scope practice within their specialty. Air Force oral and maxillofacial surgery treatment facilities range from those incorporated into large medical centers to those that are located within smaller hospital settings or dental clinics. All have access to operating rooms and inpatient facilities, whether within an Air Force medical center or regional hospital, or in some cases, at an affiliated civilian hospital in the local area.

The medical and dental needs of the large population of active-duty military beneficiaries offer ample opportunity for an abundance of experience in dentoalveolar and implant surgeries. Likewise, most Air Force oral and maxillofacial surgery practices see a wide diversity of oral pathology and maintain an ongoing need for various tumor and reconstructive surgical capabilities. Robust orthognathic surgery practices are prevalent throughout the Air Force for the treatment of functional dentofacial abnormalities and malocclusions. Opportunities also exist for facial cosmetic surgery on a fee-for-service basis.

The management of maxillofacial trauma is, of course, central to the mission of all military OMSs. Extensive craniofacial injuries are managed by Air Force OMSs in the deployed environment where a multidisciplinary approach is used. There, OMSs are working side by side with their Otolaryngology (ENT), plastic surgery, oculoplastic, and neurosurgery colleagues in the carefully coordinated management of patients with a wide variety of extensive cranial, maxillofacial, and neck injuries. Air Force OMSs are also involved in the management of maxillofacial trauma in the nondeployed setting in the treatment of active-duty personnel and other eligible beneficiaries who are injured in motor vehicle collisions, by personal assault, or as a result of participation in sports or recreational activities.

Air Force OMSs enjoy state-of-the-art facilities and the opportunity to incorporate the latest in technologic adjuncts to their practices. Digital radiography and cone-beam CT imaging is available at many Air Force oral and maxillofacial surgery clinics. Likewise, full stereolithographic modeling capabilities are readily available and are used to enhance and facilitate the treatment of cases involving extensive maxillofacial trauma, tumor and reconstructive surgeries, and craniofacial anomalies. Laser and piezoelectric surgical capabilities and hyperbaric oxygen chambers are some of the additional state-of-the-art treatment modalities available at select Air Force oral and maxillofacial surgery locations.

One of the most professionally rewarding benefits of an Air Force oral and maxillofacial surgery practice is the abundant opportunity for professional collaboration. All Air Force oral and maxillofacial surgery practices exist within a group practice setting. As previously stated, that may be in the form of a group oral and maxillofacial surgery practice itself, or within the context of a group dental practice wherein some or all of the other dental specialties are represented. Collaborative treatment planning conferences among the dental professionals at any given location is standard practice within Air Force group dental practices. Included among these conferences are dentofacial abnormalities boards and implant boards. Further collaborative opportunities exist as many Air Force OMSs function alongside their medical colleagues as integral members of craniofacial anomalies, sleep medicine, and head and neck tumor boards.

Opportunities are also available to collaborate with local civilian medical and dental professionals. Many Air Force OMSs participate in local continuing education symposia and function as members of local journal clubs and professional societies within the civilian community. Additionally, the proximity of some AFBs to civilian residency programs offers the opportunity to become involved as associate faculty members of these programs.

Obtaining board certification is emphasized within all the USAF Dental Corps, and oral and maxillofacial surgery is no exception. In the history of Air Force oral and maxillofacial surgery, 95% of all eligible practitioners have achieved diplomate status with the American Board of Oral and Maxillofacial Surgery while on active duty. Every opportunity is extended to Air Force OMSs in the pursuit of becoming board certified, including the opportunity to attend board review courses and, when available, funding to support the costs associated with taking the board examinations. Likewise, professional growth and maintaining currency is an area of emphasis for all Air Force dental officers and, toward that ideal, opportunities are extended, whenever possible, to attend national meetings and continuing education courses.

Each year, the Air Force Dental Education Committee meets to consider applications for the various postgraduate dental training programs. Among these is an opportunity for Air Force OMSs to be selected for fellowship training. Once selected for this Air Force–sponsored training, the individual has the opportunity to make formal application to accredited oral and maxillofacial surgery fellowship opportunities throughout the country. Recent fellowship opportunities extended to Air Force OMSs have included advanced training in the areas of facial cosmetic surgery, temporomandibular joint disorders and orofacial pain, and tumor and reconstructive surgery.

Air Force OMSs enjoy all the benefits of being active-duty military members, including professional liability coverage, medical and dental health care, and access to base exchange (department store) and commissary (grocery) shopping. In addition, each base location offers various other recreational opportunities, often in keeping with its particular location, such as skiing, boating, scuba and snorkeling, and travel opportunities at a discounted rate. Extensive travel opportunities abound throughout the Air Force, particularly at the overseas duty locations.

Active-duty members and their families are moved to their assigned duty locations at the expense of the Air Force. Housing opportunities exist on most AFBs and, in most cases, Air Force dental officers are given the choice of accepting on-base housing or a basic allowance for housing so that they can rent or purchase a home off base in the local area.

Summary

As described, careers as OMSs in the Federal Services have several common, yet many unique, aspects. This fulfilling and personally rewarding career has something to offer every OMS. It comes down to finding the best fit for each particular surgeon. Solo practice, small group, or large group practice is all within reach. The OMS has the ability to experiment with each setting without many of the personal or financial concerns that surface within private practice, providing a significant opportunity for the OMS with a sense of, or yearning for, service to country. Whether it is education, clinical, research, leadership, or administrative, the opportunity for each, some, or all is there in the Federal Services. The interested OMS simply needs to reach out, get on board, hold on, and enjoy the ride of a professional lifetime. This life opportunity is there for the taking.

How to Plan a Successful Associateship and Practice Transition

Stanley L. Pollock, BS, DMD, MS, PhD, JD

Professional Practice Planners, 332 5th Avenue, Suite 213, McKeesport, PA 15132, USA

Associate—a work partner or colleague. Associateship—being connected with a colleague, business, or professional practice—the major form of the oral & maxillofacial surgery practice today, and the significant subject of this chapter. Over the years, the number of oral & maxillofacial surgeons practicing in some form of associateship has increased tremendously. In the 1960s that percentage was around 27%; today it is more than 65%. There are multiple reasons for this significant 140% plus increase. Such reasons are, but not limited to, starting or prolonging a career; relieving an excessive patient load; making personal and professional lives simpler and easier; initiating new procedures, techniques and methods; creating new and reviving stalled markets; enhancing mutual consultations and in-office peer review; sharing certain practice expenses; expanding scope of services, practices, and opportunities; merging; and, importantly, finding and creating a buyer or buyers of the practice.[1]

The typical oral & maxillofacial surgeon completing advanced training programs is heavily in debt and is either unable or unwilling to incur the sizeable debt service required to enter private oral & maxillofacial surgery practice. Rather, she/he is more eager to start paying down the incurred, heavy debt. Additionally, the many oral & maxillofacial surgeons leaving the various military and public health services and academia are eager to settle down and put their talents into private practice. There are multiple types of associateships, which include employee–employer, independent contractor–employer, time–space–expense sharing, owner–partner, and partnership of corporations/business entity. Each has certain characteristics, advantages, and disadvantages. In this chapter, we focus on the equity type in which (1) an oral & maxillofacial surgeon joins a practice as an associate, (2) becomes a minor equity owner, and (3) eventually becomes an equal and major principal in the organization.

The general associateship process, from neophyte to equity owner to departing partner, comprises three phases—trial, buy-in, and buy-out. This article encompasses these three phases. It is imperative, however, that readers thoroughly comprehend and embrace the panoptic concept and fact that an associateship is a complex process. It is imperative that each doctor, whether senior or one anticipating to be an associate, do a great deal of veritable self-searching and analysis, have or put a team in place, and discuss the various and crucial matters with the team. Although the entire team may not be involved initially, the team initially will consist of an accountant, attorney, and appraiser. Later, a banker, practice management consultant, realtor, insurance professional, and financial planner may become involved. All should be professionally competent and experienced in professional practice transitions. For an associateship of any type to succeed, the entire process must be well planned, flexible, and properly initiated and monitored. Otherwise, the associateship is doomed to fail!

If the form of the practice at this stage has been a solo proprietorship, it will become necessary, and this is a good time to change the business form to either a form of partnership (limited

---

E-mail address: stanpoll@aol.com

[1] Practice –> practice, business entity, corporation, general partnership, limited liability company, and partnerships are used throughout and are interchangeable whether two-doctor or multi-doctor.

liability company, general partnership, limited partnership) or corporation (C or S types). After discussions with her/his accountant or attorney with regard to the advantages and disadvantages of each form, Doctor Senior selects the most practical form of business enterprise.

Analysis–evaluation–considerations

The associate

Today, oral & maxillofacial surgeons are very mobile. They travel to distant universities, graduate from dental and medical schools, and continue all over the United States to complete advanced oral & maxillofacial and facial surgery programs. Many come from Canada and foreign countries and eventually remain in the United States. Green cards are common today. Many states have eased their licensing requirements and others permit and encourage licensing by credentials.

An oral & maxillofacial surgeon anticipating an associateship must consider the following factors:

1. Will I be able to practice the scope of oral & maxillofacial surgery for which I have been trained, prefer, and enjoy?
2. Will my family and I enjoy living and participating in the community?
3. Are suitable educational, religious, and health care facilities available?
4. Are environmental, climate, and recreational factors favorable?
5. Is suitable, reasonable housing available?
6. What is the general cost of living in the community?
7. Is suitable employment available for my spouse or significant other?
8. What is the overall tax structure in the community?
9. Is shopping convenient?
10. Will we be too distant or too close to family?
11. Do I or my family require any special needs?
12. Do I genuinely believe I am a "team" player and "group" oriented?
13. Others?

The senior oral & maxillofacial surgeon

1. Is the patient load adequate? Increasing? Decreasing? Steady? Why?
2. Do patients have to wait an inordinate amount of time to obtain treatment?
3. Does the practice's financial condition warrant an associate?
4. Can/will the practice afford an associate?
5. Am I truly willing and expect to share, teach, change, and learn? Am I psychologically prepared and adjusted?
6. Am I truly willing to give up certain control?
7. Do I have a competent, experienced team in place?
8. Have I consulted with my team members?
9. Is the present facility adequate?
10. Will I have to enlarge my staff?
11. Will I have to or do I plan to expand or refurbish?
12. Will I have to purchase new or additional equipment?
13. Others?

Preparation

General

It is crucial that parties forming and entering in an associateship with implied partnership/ownership understand the relationship shall be long term. The initial term is important, but the long-term consequences are even more important. On a sheet of paper or two, each doctor should consider and write a MISSION STATEMENT. The mission statement should be a clear and succinct representation of the professional enterprise and each individual's participation in the enterprise. The intent should be a powerful, initial consideration. To remove all third molars in the community is a grand but unrealistic mission statement. Simply, the mission statement realistically encompasses what the parties are trying to accomplish in a professional environment.

Each party must sincerely write down her/his GOALS AND OBJECTIVES. This is highly crucial for the parties' goals, and objectives, in general, must blend. They cannot blend, however, until each party truly knows what they are and freely discusses them with each other. Goals and objectives can range from simple to complex, from moderate to extreme, from personal to entity effective; yet the must be pragmatic and workable. Unless the parties understand their goals and objectives, they cannot discuss them, much less accomplish them. The parties must consider where they are today and where they would like to be in a year, in 5 years, and in 10 years.

Obviously, the Doctors have EXPECTATIONS AND CONCERNS. Doctor Senior may anticipate retiring in a few years or providing extensive missionary services. Doctor Junior may expect to become an equal owner in a year or so, which may or may not be feasible. Doctor Senior may have had a previous associate, and Doctor Junior may have been an associate previously, and, for whatever reason, the associateships did not work out. The doctors may be of different religious backgrounds, which, certainly, requires discussion, education, and accommodation. These and others would be major concerns, and the doctors should be aware of and openly discuss these and other matters to allay their concerns. Open discussion of any and all expectations and concerns is healthy and will go a long way to achieving a successful associateship.

Planning and forming an associateship is not inexpensive. Each doctor will incur costs and, therefore, should prepare a budget to cover the costs. Box 1 provides a reasonable estimate of such costs. It is imperative that Doctor Senior have the practice entity realistically valued before the associate's entry. All parties involved with the entire process should know the true value of the entity. Each will want to know how much it will cost Doctor Junior to buy in to the entity and how she or he will pay it at the appropriate time. Not having a realistic valuation in place has been the major reason that associateships break up. Not only will the pre-associateship valuation prevent many major problems, but it will also serve as a feasibility study, make cash flow projections, and present pertinent ratios. The valuation or appraisal form the crucial basis involved in the buy-in, compensation, buy-sell agreement and pay-out. At the very least, this aspect commands frank discussion early in the process.

Finally, structuring an associateship is not a do-it-yourself project. Although the Doctors must and will have to do a great deal of the ground work, they require the expertise of competent, experienced, support advisors. As stated, each doctor requires and shall lead a team, but the team must be in place.

Preparation

Senior oral & maxillofacial surgeon

1. Meet and discuss matters with consultants.
2. Understand basic financial factors, such as gross and net revenues and true operational expenses.
3. Prepare "fact pact" or "associate's terms"—the Package (Box 2).
4. Obtain realistic practice valuation/appraisal from a competent, certified professional practice appraiser.
5. Understand that it will probably cost between $10,000 and $20,000 to bring an associate on board—prepare a budget (see Box 1).
6. Determine cost of package for initial term of associate (Box 3).

Preparation considerations

Junior oral & maxillofacial surgeon

1. Consider location and other above-listed factors.
2. Prepare résumé/curriculum vitae with cover letter.
3. Prepare and check advertisements.
4. Consider reasonable compensation and/or incentive compensation.
5. Consider benefits: initial and renewal terms (Box 4).
6. Consider advancement: equity ownership and position.
7. Seek competent, experienced advisors (the "team").
8. Prepare budget.
9. Consider additional factors.

It is manifestly evident that comprehensive preparation is crucial to any associateship. Not infrequently, in preparatory planning, certain factors show up that reveal that an associate and associateship are not indicated or feasible at the time. This is extremely valuable for planning, because entering an unwarranted associateship would be disastrous, and all parties could be

---

Box 1. Cost estimate to commence associateship process

1. Initial consultations, $1000
2. Comprehensive valuation, $3000+++
3. Advertising, $1000
4. Recruiting: interviews, etc, $5000
5. Employment agreement, letter of intent, $1250
6. Miscellaneous $1000
TOTAL $12,250+

> **Box 2. The "fact pact" – associateship terms – dream sheet**
>
> 1. Status: employee of practice (sole proprietorship, corporation, partnership, limited liability company or partnership
> 2. Term: 12 months with automatic renewal (60-day termination clause for either party without cause and/or liability)
> 3. Restrictive covenants, antisolicitation clauses (24 months and reasonable radius from any office)
> 4. Compensation: $ _____ per year with/without incentive compensation or bonus (includes allocation and allowance for consideration of covenants)
> 5. Benefits:
>   a. Professional liability insurance (malpractice): should it be required before associate's buy-in phase, associate shall immediately obtain and pay for the so-called "tail coverage"
>   b. Health care benefits: provided associate is not rated or covered under another's benefit program
>   c. Professional dues, licenses, DEA certificate, staff applications: as selected and approved, annual, in full or up to a specific amount
>   d. Continuing education, vacation, sick leave: 3 weeks with specific allowance for continuing education and consideration for American Board examinations
>   e. Practice to provide current facility(s), pager, cellular telephone, personnel, equipment, supplies
>   f. Social security, Medicare, unemployment, state and federal worker's compensation
> 6. At the end of initial term, provided associate's professionalism and production/collection are adequate and it is mutually agreeable, the doctors shall commence associate's becoming an equity owner of the practice entity. Doctor Senior has had the practice realistically valued before the associate's entry into the organization and shall hold that value as the buy-in commences. Doctor Senior shall prepare and present a general plan for the associate's method of buy-in of up to a 50% interest.

disappointed. On the other hand, conscientious analysis and planning will organize the parties for a comprehensive and gratifying experience.

Advertising and recruitment

Now that the doctors have managed the preliminary consultations and comprehensive preparation, they make the decision to go forward with the process. So how do the doctors know to reach each other? Simply, getting the word out—which consists of contacting reliable, experienced professional practice brokers and dental equipment and supply companies; running ads in the appropriate professional journals and AAOMS TODAY (the American Association of Oral & Maxillofacial Surgery bimonthly publication);

> **Box 3. Cost of associate's "package"**
>
> Base salary, $150,000
> Incentive compensation, $10,000
> Social security + Medicare, $8210
> Malpractice insurance, $4000
> Health care–family, $10,000
> Continuing education, $2500
> Dues, licenses, applications $2500
> Cell phone, pager $1200
> Additional: stationery, cards, signage, etc, $2500
> TOTAL, $190,910
> Consider: increased personnel, additional equipment, relocation expense, expansion, refurbishing, others
> $190,910 ÷ 47% (NET PROFIT PERCENT) = *$406,191* = BREAKEVEN POINT
> Practice shall require approximately $400,000 new or increased revenues to *break even* with regard to associate's compensation and benefits.

> **Box 4. Benefits**
>
> 1. Malpractice insurance
> 2. Health care insurance
> 3. Life insurance
> 4. Disability income insurance
> 5. Dental insurance/care
> 6. Medical reimbursement
> 7. Vehicle: lease, ownership
> 8. Vehicle: expense, maintenance
> 9. Dues
> 10. Licenses
> 11. Hospital and other applications
> 12. Subscriptions, publications
> 13. Moving, relocation
> 14. Telephone: cellular telephone, pager
> 15. Child, parent, family care
> 16. Travel
> 17. Pension plan contributions
> 18. Profit sharing plan contributions
> 19. Promotion, entertainment
> 20. Vacation with pay
> 21. Continuing education, board preparation
> 22. Personal days with pay
> 23. Legal and accounting
> 24. Sick leave with pay
> 25. Financial, estate, other planning
> 26. Leave of absence with/without pay
> 27. Uniforms, uniform allowance
> 28. Textbooks, library
> 29. Vision care
> 30. Pharmaceuticals
> 31. Club membership and expenses, health, country, city
> 32. Other

contacting chairpersons of the training programs; sending and posting notices to the training programs; and word of mouth. Junior doctors will also mail notices to selected practitioners and run selected ads. Many doctors prefer to remain anonymous, which is okay and which is possible; these doctors use box numbers or practice consultants.

Action

It is important to understand that each oral & maxillofacial surgeon, each oral & maxillofacial surgery practice, and each associate and associateship are unique and wonderful. Each associateship, then, is, and should be, customized for the participants. Accordingly, the actions and activities shall be general in nature. The doctors shall understand, agree to, and sign a written covenant that all personal and professional discussions and exchange of information and tax and financial data, including work product, are extremely confidential; they shall not disclose any information to any individual or outside source other than close and active professional advisors who shall, similarly, agree to this confidential covenant unless they have the others' written permission or are required by law.

When the parties screen and respond to the advertised sources, Doctor Senior shall contact Doctor Junior and arrange the first interview. Normally, this should take around one hour in the office and is a "meeting of the minds." Over lunch, normally, is inadequate. This is the time when the doctors exchange ideas relative to their mission statements, goals, objectives, expectations, and concerns. Doctor Senior presents Doctor Junior with the "fact pact," explains it is a "package," and briefly discusses the items included in the package. Doctor Senior advises Doctor Junior to review the fact pact with his advisor so they can discuss it at the next session. Chances are the meeting will end with each doctor's advising, if indeed this is the case, that she/he has other interviews lined up, and they will contact each other shortly for the next interview.

If the interview has gone well, and each doctor was impressed with the other, they take the next step, the second interview. This interview should be scheduled for a full day, and Doctor Senior should modify his schedule appropriately. Doctor Senior shows Doctor Junior the office, introduces her or him to the staff, and shows Doctor Junior how he and the staff operate. They may go together to the hospital or ambulatory care center and, in general, Doctor Senior introduces Doctor Junior to the private practice of oral & maxillofacial surgery. They hold frank discussions over lunch or dinner and at the end of the day, they discuss those issues particularly related to their goals, expectations, concerns, licensing, the American Board of Oral & Maxillofacial Surgery, and the fact pact. Hopefully, the doctors leave in good spirits and arrange to meet again shortly.

After further discussion with their advisors, the doctors arrange a third interview which may encompass a complete day or more. If appropriate, the spouse or significant other joins Doctor Junior, and Doctor Senior's spouse accompanies her/him on a trip around the community. Major areas are housing, shopping, schools, health care, places of worship, and other facilities. The doctors spend productive time in the office. Doctor Senior offers Doctor Junior an associateship position, reviews the agreed-upon terms of the fact pact, and advises that his attorney shall send him a detailed Employment Agreement based on the agreed-upon fact pact. Doctor Junior soon receives the agreement and, along with his attorney, reviews it, possibly makes minimal revisions, and signs the agreement, and both doctors, then, have taken the first step to ensure their career-shaping transition.

Throughout the overall associateship process, the doctors will be under a great deal of pressure, because the process and its extensive ordeals will be unfamiliar and difficult. Most likely they will be involved and negotiating with multiple candidates, doctors, and consultants. The doctors, nevertheless, must be sincere, honest, and professional with each other. They must be highly principled and exhibit scrupulous integrity. There simply is no room for deception, misleading, ill manners, or stalling.

Phase one—trial or break-in phase

Upon the effective date, Doctor Junior and family have moved to the community, and the doctors start the associateship. Doctor Senior sends an announcement to referral sources and others that doctor Junior has joined her or him in the practice, and Doctor Junior commences an organized promotion campaign. The doctors advance throughout the initial term. They work together, educate each other, blend together, and enhance the practice. On a monthly basis, they monitor the progress in all areas, which include, but are not limited to, clinical proficiency, attitude, professional relations and communications, cooperation with management, staff relations, continuing education, attendance, and marketing. They examine Doctor Junior's commitment to time, energy, and effort to continuing and maintaining the standards of the oral & maxillofacial surgery profession and the practice. They consider Doctor Junior's productivity and effort to control overhead of the practice. They discuss what may be required to improve any deficiencies and to elevate the practice to a higher level.

Phase two—the buy-in

The relationship has progressed favorably and has been mutually rewarding. Doctor Junior's professionalism and productivity have been superior. She or he understands that hospital appointments and advancement and complete equity position in the practice entity are dependent on Doctor Junior's taking and passing the examinations of the American Board of Oral & Maxillofacial Surgery. The doctors take measures to encourage and accommodate Doctor Junior's Board certification. Phase two is the phase in which Doctor Junior commences becoming an equity owner in the practice entity. Doctor Senior had the entity valued before Doctor Junior's entry into the organization and maintains that value. She or he also has a general plan in place for Doctor Junior's buy-in, which the dDoctors shall now implement.

In this case and as an illustration, the fair market value of 100% of the value of the stock and interest in the Corporation is $500,000. The value of the 50% interest that Doctor Junior shall purchase, of course, is $250,000. The term of the normal buy-in is 5 years, although the term may vary from 3 to 8 or even 10 years. Doctor Senior breaks down the 50% interest into the following portions and values:

Tangible Asset Value (Stock or Unit)	*$75,000*
Intangible Asset Value (Goodwill, Going Concern)	*$175,000*

The Internal Revenue Service (IRS) requires and Doctor Junior shall purchase and pay for her or his stock or unit purchase.[2] Doctor Junior, then, shall pay Doctor Senior $15,000 annually or $1250 per month during the term of the buy-in. Doctor Junior shall purchase her/his stock from Doctor Senior in the same manner that she or he shall purchase any stock from a friendly broker. At the end of each year when Doctor Junior has paid Doctor Senior in full, Doctor Senior shall issue to Doctor Junior a certificate for her/his ten percent interest in the entity so that at the end of the five year term, the Doctors shall each have a fifty percent interest in the organization.

---

[2] *Stock* is used in the case of the entity's being a corporation; *unit*, if the entity is a limited liability company in full, Doctor Senior shall issue Dr. Junior a certificate for her/his 10% interest in the entity so that at the end of the 5-year term, the doctors shall each have a 50% interest in the organization.

Years ago, for a Senior Doctor to maintain "control" of the practice, Doctor Senior would sell Doctor Junior only up to 49% of her/his stock. This is not so common today, for Doctor Senior can still maintain "control" by having certain clauses in various entity agreements, which, in case of a tie in voting, her/his vote would be superior and break any such tie. Other stipulations such as noncancellable employment and leaves of absence can be built into the practice's agreements.

The doctors agree that Doctor Junior shall pay for her/his intangible asset portion on an income adjustment basis. Doctor Junior shall receive a certain amount LESS each month, and Doctor Senior shall receive a similar amount MORE each month. Normally, the annual amount would be $35,000, and Doctor Senior would pay the tax on the gain of her/his sale for his entire purchases at her/his long-term capital gain rate, which currently is 15%. However, because the intangible portion shall be adjusted or shifted to Doctor Senior, she/he shall be taxed at much higher combined federal and state ordinary tax rates—around 40%. The difference, of course, between the two rates is 25%, and this difference shall be, similarly, adjusted or shifted to Doctor Junior's intangible purchase. The annual $35,000 times the 25% difference becomes $43,750, Accordingly, Doctor Junior shall adjust or shift to Doctor Senior $3,646 per month for her/his intangible asset purchase. For the above transactions, the doctors require stock or unit purchase, individual employment, and administrative agreements.

The doctors also must have a comprehensive buy–sell agreement in place for equal partners. This agreement simply directs conditions concerning when and how a doctor who is an equal or greater owner departs from the organization in case of premature death and permanent disability, retirement, and all other voluntary and involuntary reasons and when, how, and how much she/he shall receive. If the associate departs from the practice during her/his buy-in phase, for any reason, the practice entity or senior doctor shall repurchase his stock or units, normally, at a reduced amount and in the same time frame that Doctor Junior purchased her/his stock or units and shall include interest.

Occasionally, the doctors will decide that they become equal owners (50:50) of the entity at the beginning of the buy-in term. Doctor Junior, then, shall pay Doctor Senior $75,000 at the beginning of the term. She/he would obtain funding from a relative or spouse or either float a third party loan, or Doctor Senior would finance the purchase. In the latter two cases, because Doctor Junior is receiving her/his stock or interest initially, the IRS requires the loan be assessed a reasonable interest rate. The doctors shall still structure the intangible portion adjusted purchase over 5 years. What is important to understand in this overall financing process is that (1) Doctor Junior shall receive her/his tangible and intangible basis on an interest-free basis, (2) Doctor Junior, normally, does not have to obtain bank or third party financing, and (3) the practice entity shall provide Doctor Junior with adequate compensation to pay for her/his buy-in.

Compensation

Compensation is pertinent to the success of an associateship. It is also pertinent for the doctors to understand that compensation and ownership are two distinct features and not necessarily related to each other. There are myriad methods for income sharing, probably as many as the number of associateships. All fall under a few general approaches. Proper determination of compensation requires realistic cash flow projections based on past results with consideration for gross revenues; overhead; taxes; future expenditures of equipment, furniture, and improvements; determined income adjustments; and others. The approaches relate to division of net income and are, but not limited to:

Equal
Production/collection percentage
Production percentage less expense percentage
Production less allocation of expenses
Equal percentage/production percentage
Fixed salary—associate
Fixed salary with incentive—associate
Percent of senior partner's income
Additional

Equal

This is the oldest and simplest method and not as common as in the past. After deducting expenses, the doctors equally split the net income and add and subtract the income adjustments.

Production/collection percentage

Each surgeon's compensation is based on the total revenues that she/he produces and the practice entity collects as a percentage of total revenues. Should Doctor Senior produce 65% of the collected revenues, she/he would receive 65% of the net income plus the income adjustment. Doctor Junior would receive 35% of the net income less the income adjustment.

Production/collection percentage less expense percentage

This method is similar to the previous method except that each surgeon is responsible and deducts the same percentage of the true operational expenses. If Doctor Senior produced 65% of the collected revenues, Doctor Senior would be responsible for 65% of the true operational expenses. Similarly, if Doctor Junior produced 35% of the collected revenues, Doctor Junior would be responsible for 35% of the true operational expenses. In this method, adjustments are appropriately added and subtracted.

Equal percentage/production percentage

This method is an attempt to equalize certain differences in income division and to account for unequal division of cases and time. Each surgeon's compensation is based on (1) a percentage of the net income divided equally and (2) a percentage of the net income divided based on her/his personal production/collection as a percentage of the total collected revenues. Percentages run from 50%/50% to 80%/20% generally. Of course, income adjustments are appropriately added and subtracted.

Fixed salary—associate

In this method, the associate simply receives an annual fixed reduced salary without subtraction of the income adjustment, which is considered in the determination of fixed salary.

Fixed salary with incentive—associate

This method is similar to the above method, but an incentive is built in that is based on the percentage of the associate's collections over a predetermined benchmark or break-even amount.

Percentage of the senior partner's income

This method is used when the entity's value is not specifically determined, and the surgeons simply are satisfied to divide income on Doctor Junior's annual increasing percentage. Annual percentages vary from 40% to 60% initially with increases of 10% until the income is divided equally. These fixed salary and annual increasing percentage methods are indirect or inexact methods, primarily used in large revenue organizations, and eliminate specific income adjustments.

Additional

Other methods of compensation are based on the number of days worked and consideration for taking or not taking after-hours calls and reasonable additional compensation for a surgeon's providing management services after normal operating hours. Although the normal timeframe for buy-ins today is 5 years, depending on the realistic valuation of the professional entity and the gross and net incomes, the time frame may be extended or reduced. When an associate becomes an equal entity owner, the doctors determine the method of compensation without the adjustments. The doctors can alter their method of compensation whenever they feel it is appropriate. At all times, they may and must regard the fixed, variable, and direct expenses in their compensation considerations.

Benefits

Benefits, which can number from 30 to 35 (see Box 4), play a large part in the doctors' overall compensation and satisfaction. The associate's benefits are reasonable during the first and second phases and increase annually until the doctors reach parity. At the same time, certain direct benefits are allocated and considered in each doctor's total compensation. There, simply, is no "one right" way to determine compensation. There are myriad factors that require personal and professional consideration, deliberate analysis, and consultation with proficient advisors and, sometimes, experimentation.

Phase three—the buy-out

As stated above, phase three is the phase in which a senior doctor shall depart from the active practice of oral & maxillofacial surgery. The doctors have been practicing together and achieving a great deal professionally, personally, and community-wise. The Associateship has been well planned and successful. Doctor Senior had previously advised Doctor Junior, who is Junior only by her/his time in service with the organization now, that at age 65 he would retire from active practice. He is one year from his stated goal and has given Doctor Junior written notice of her/his intent to retire.

At the beginning of phase two, the doctors had prepared and have in place a comprehensive buysell agreement. This important document states in specific format when and how an equal partner may/shall depart in all cases—premature death and permanent disability, retirement and voluntary and involuntary reasons. Importantly, the document describes how much a departing Doctor shall receive upon departure and when she/he shall receive it as well as in what form (Box 5). The buy-sell agreement also states that the doctors shall review the terms of the agreement, more particularly, the valuation of the tangible and intangible assets, annually.

The buy-out method resembles and mirrors the buy-in and breaks down into two major portions, the tangible or stock or unit portion and intangible or goodwill portion. The agreement states how the tangible portion shall be calculated and recorded, which, again, is tied into the fair market values of the tangible or fixed assets. Subtracting the tangible asset value from the total value results in the intangible or goodwill and covenant not to compete values. The buy-sell agreement and arrangements are necessary and constitute a business continuation plan.

Funding of the terms of the buy-sell agreement is vital. Fortunately, insurance is available to help fund the pay-out of a departing doctor. Various forms of life insurance, with and without cash surrender values, and disability buy-out and business interruption insurance favor premature death and disability events. Key-person, split dollar, term, and other types of insurance abound today at reasonable cost albeit expensive. Disability income insurance is definitely important and requires consideration. Buying insurance, determining the right kind, deciding how much is actually necessary, and knowing the countless riders and terms can be confusing. Engaging the services of a competent insurance professional, perhaps, will alleviate the multiple problems.

In our case, Doctor Senior has given written one year's notice of his retirement and guarantee not to practice oral & maxillofacial surgery in the geographic area. The notice gives Doctor Junior a year to find a suitable, competent associate, and the parties shall follow the general outline and the three-phase method that is in place. The numbers, most likely, will be different, but the methodology will be the same.

At the end of the year, Doctor Senior shall receive any compensation due and shall repay any loans incurred. Normally, the accounts receivable and payable and liabilities are included in the valuation. The practice entity, Doctor Junior, or new associate shall purchase Doctor Senior's stock or units and his goodwill and covenant not to compete. He/she shall pay at least 10% upon departure and the remainder plus reasonable interest over 5 years. At this date, Doctor Senior will pay taxes on his stock/unit and goodwill pay-out at his long-term capital gain rate of 15% and for his covenant not to compete and interest at his ordinary tax rate as received. If Doctor Junior has been unable to find Doctor Right, Doctor Senior may work part time as an independent contractor oral & maxillofacial surgeon.

Two final points

Regardless of the form of associateship, it is imperative that the doctors commit the terms and accords to detailed written agreements. Handshakes are great, but memories are not. Written agreements help avoid misunderstandings and confusion, particularly, in the future when memories may fail.

Throughout the phases and at all times, bailouts are necessary and must be built into the terms of all agreements. Philosophies, goals, and

---

Box 5. Terms of the buy-sell agreement

1. Parties
2. Effective date
3. Background
4. Transfer of shares to non-shareholder/member
5. Obligation to purchase upon premature death
6. Insurance
7. Obligation to purchase upon permanent disability
8. Retirement: terms and obligation to purchase
9. Agreed "price," the valuation, reviews
10. Obligation to purchase upon other events
11. Method of payment
12. Security
13. Postretirement employment
14. Additional

attitudes, unfortunately, change and require accommodation.

Summary

We have covered a great of material relative to planning and implementing an associateship. We started with the reasons for, types of, and basic concepts involved with an associateship. We focused on an oral & maxillofacial surgeon's decision to become an associate and an oral & maxillofacial surgeon's decision to accept an associate into her/his practice and becoming an equal equity owner ("partner, shareholder, member") in the practice entity. The doctors, naturally, have specific and general goals, objectives, motives, visions, concerns, expectations, and considerations requiring detailed analyses and evaluation that they must address. They must be willing to teach, learn, and share control. They must have compatible understandings and philosophies because most associateships are long term. They require competent advisors and a budget. They must have a realistic valuation and mutual, understandable written and unwritten agreements. We showed, once the doctors decide to plan and form an associateship, the general process of advertising, recruiting, interviewing, and accepting an associate. We separated and illustrated the process into three phases. We concluded that not only must the doctors be willing to devote a great deal of time and effort to building the practice but even greater time and effort into building and nurturing the associateship.

Key points

1. Confidentiality, sincerity, honesty and professionalism are paramount.
2. Understand the process—be prepared.
3. Allow sufficient time for the process and phases.
4. Communicate at the highest level—keep it open—but do *not* stall.
5. Consult and work with qualified, experienced individuals.
6. An associateship is a serious, career-shaping business—"don't play games."
7. Look at the overall "big picture"—no place for pettiness.
8. Think: where do I/we want to be in a year? 5 years? 10 years?
9. Don't try to squeeze every drop out of every situation.
10. Remember—generally, an associateship is "long term."
11. Normally, covenants are necessary as long as they are reasonable (Box 6).
12. Memories fade, so commit the results of your discussions and decisions to reasonable, understandable legal writing.
13. Understand: someone started the practice, nurtured it, and raised it to the associate level.

Box 6. Restrictive covenants

1. Fall under each state's statutes and case law
2. Recognized by some—not recognized by few others
3. Regardless, must
   a. be reasonable in length of time (24 months most common today)
   b. be reasonable in geographic area
   c. not be unduly harsh or oppressive
   d. not be harmful to public interest
   e. not be greater than necessary to protect legitimate interest of party. (*Data from* Karpinsky v. Ignasci, 268 NE 2d 751 [1971]).
4. Factors:
   a. must include "consideration" in agreement
   b. cannot deny "right to work" and "restraint of trade"
   c. liquidated damages
5. Normally, restrictive covenants will stand up if above guideline followed

Common Contractual Concerns for the Oral and Maxillofacial Surgeon

Eugene W. Luciani, JD

Anderson, Tate & Carr, P.C., 1505 Lakes Parkway, Suite 100, Lawrenceville, GA 30043, USA

The oral and maxillofacial surgeon ("OMS") faces varied and complex issues on a daily basis. Usually, these are matters for which the OMS has had extensive training and practice. Whether new to private practice or a seasoned practitioner, an OMS will need to understand how to handle complicated and often stressful negotiations of contracts for which the OMS usually is untrained. This article is designed to give the OMS a general understanding of certain common contractual language. This article is not comprehensive in scope but rather attempts to cover contracts that are most often seen by an OMS in his or her practice.

Letters of intent

Parties use letters of intent (LOIs) to set the groundwork for formal agreements and to ensure the parties have the same general understanding of the basic terms of a deal before significant costs and expenses are incurred in drafting lengthy agreements. LOIs often appear as letters but sometimes can appear as more formal legal documents. LOIs generally are characterized by their nonbinding nature with respect to the substantive business terms mentioned in such letter.

OMSs most often see LOIs in the context of associateships and buy-ins. An OMS and a practice must consider numerous concerns when going to work as or hiring a new associate OMS. Once the parties have weighed these factors and decided have that the OMS would make a good associate, the existing practice or the senior doctor usually will ask his/her lawyers to prepare a LOI or, in some instances, an employment agreement (as discussed later). A LOI usually has a nonbinding section and a binding section.

The nonbinding section typically contains the basic business terms of the proposed transaction. In the context of employment, the nonbinding section of the LOI normally contains information on the proposed salary, bonus structure, benefits, duration, and criteria for being made a partner/shareholder/member of the practice, whether the practice will pay for moving expenses, and the anticipated start date of the associate OMS. (The terms "partner," "shareholder," and "member" are used to represent a status of, or a person holding, an equity ownership in a partnership [general or limited], a corporation, or a limited liability company [LLC], respectively).

Usually these employment terms become binding only when the parties agree to a definitive, separate employment agreement containing the terms. Generally speaking, the LOI is not a document that either party should expect to be able to enforce against the other with respect to the items in the nonbinding section.

The binding portions of the LOI usually contain confidentiality provisions. The practice may want to show the potential new employee OMS certain trade secrets, its future plans for growth and expansion, and certain techniques the practice may feel are proprietary. Naturally, the practice needs to protect these valuable aspects of its business, so the parties customarily agree to a reasonable confidentiality provision in LOIs.

The author is a shareholder in Andersen, Tate & Carr, P.C., a general practice law firm in Lawrenceville, Georgia.

This is not, nor is it intended to be, legal advice. Each person should consult his/her own attorney for advice regarding such person's individual situation.

E-mail address: gluciani@atclawfirm.com

The confidentiality provision also may require the potential employee OMS to keep the terms of the deal confidential; however, the employee OMS should insist on an exception that allows him/her to discuss the deal's terms with his/her financial advisors, accountants, and lawyers. In addition, the practice may request that the potential employee OMS not seek alternative employment for a certain period of time while the practice spends time and money drafting a definitive employment agreement and possibly a buy-in agreement after the LOI is signed. If both parties agree to such a provision, the employee OMS should consider asking for a reciprocal clause wherein the practice would not seek another employee or negotiate with another potential associate for the position that prospective employee OMS would occupy. These exclusive negotiation terms do not appear in all LOIs but do give the parties a period of time during which they know that they will deal with only one another and will negotiate in good faith to come to a formal, definitive agreement.

Although LOIs provide a fairly informal means by which the parties can set out their general understanding of a deal, they do have difficulties and problems. The informal nature of these documents often lulls unsuspecting parties into either unexpectedly creating binding obligations prematurely or agreeing to items they did not understand to be part of the deal. Often lawyers see a previously signed LOI that a client claims is nonbinding that in fact has every element of a binding contract. As with any legal document, it is imperative that LOIs be written and reviewed by a lawyer. Many litigation attorneys correctly believe that LOIs are fertile ground for expensive litigation because parties spend too little time and attention in making sure that these informal documents do not do more than the parties really intended. For this reason alone, many lawyers advise clients to skip the LOI stage and move directly to the negotiation of formal agreements containing the definitive terms of the deal. In summary, LOIs can be an economical means to ensure the basic understanding of the deal is consistent among the parties; however, the OMS should never take LOIs casually, even though their informal nature may tempt one to do so.

Employment agreements

The associate employment agreement is probably the most important document a new OMS will negotiate when entering into private practice. This one document will contain the binding terms related to how much the OMS will earn, what kind of benefits he/she will receive, how much vacation he/she will receive, and of course how many days he/she will take call. Although all of these items are negotiable, the major terms of the employment agreement such as salary, vacation, call, and bonus should be discussed and generally understood before the employment agreement is drafted If the parties used an LOI, the LOIs should contain those terms. If the parties did not use an LOI, these essential terms should be discussed and agreed to in detail by the OMS and the practice before the lawyers are given their drafting assignments. Spending time negotiating essential business terms while negotiating the legal language in the employment agreement can lead only to frustration, anxiety, and bad feelings between the parties. No one wants to start a relationship this way.

Compensation

Of course, when the OMS receives the employment agreement, his/her first priority should be making sure that the business terms are properly reflected in the document. The employment agreement must contain clear, unambiguous language about how to calculate the salary (if it is not a fixed amount) and how and when bonus amounts are to be paid. Compensation structures and bonus structures for OMSs can be very complicated. When negotiating these terms, an OMS must keep in mind that although the language may make sense to him/her, it also must make sense to a judge or jury. Clear, concise formulas should be used in favor of general concepts. For example, if the OMS will obtain a percentage of certain profits, the revenues and costs that make up the "profits" should be defined precisely. Simply saying "profits" or "net profits" may mean one thing to the OMS and another to the practice, thereby causing considerable dissention (and possibly litigation) at bonus time.

Term and termination

Generally, associate employment agreements run for a 12-month period and are renewed automatically for successive 12-month periods unless one party gives notice to the other that it does not want to renew. Most agreements also allow the practice to terminate an associate's employment for "cause" and allow either party to terminate "without cause." The distinction between "cause" and "without cause" is critical, because a termination for cause by the employer may cost the employee his/her bonus and also could lead to a reduction in the price of stock or units to be bought back from an employee shareholder or member. (The term "shares" is used to indicate ownership in a corporation, and the term "units" is used to indicate ownership in an LLC or partnership, although ownership interests in partnerships and LLCs actually may be referred to by other terms.)

Although there is no standard definition of "cause," an example of language defining "cause" is as follows:

> "Cause" shall be any of the following:
> (1) Employee's permanent disqualification from practicing medicine or suspension of Employee's medical license by the [State Board of Medical Examiners]; (2) Employee's death or disability [which will need to be defined in the agreement]; (3) Employee's use of illegal substances; (4) inability of Employer to reasonably obtain malpractice insurance on Employee due to Employee's acts or omissions; (5) involuntary termination of Employee's staff privileges for more than thirty (30) consecutive days (other than for failure to complete medical records) at any hospital where Employee regularly admits or treats patients; (6) violation by Employee of any material term or condition of this Employment Agreement, including but not limited to Employee's repeated failure (after written notice) to complete Employer's patient medical records, which is not cured within thirty (30) calendar days after written notice of the breach is given; (7) Employee's conviction or plea of guilty to a felony or any crime of fraud involving patients, payors, or a governmental entity; (8) Employee's proven commission of an act of fraud within Employer's practice, or act of proven malpractice, or misfeasance, or dishonesty, or any other act which is materially detrimental to Employer or any of its patients; (9) impairment in performing duties by use of alcohol or drugs; or (10) participation in business unrelated to Employer which creates substantial conflict with the Employee's full-time practice with Employer.

This language indicates the types of acts that may constitute cause and allow the employer to terminate the employee immediately or, in some instances, on 30 days' notice. Although other language may be substituted, and other concerns may be added or deleted, it is important that the employee negotiate out any subjective criteria from the definition of "cause." For example, some employment agreements contain a morals clause providing that employee can be terminated with cause if he/she engages in immoral conduct or commits actions that negatively affect the reputation of the practice. These morals clauses are inherently subjective and could be abused by one party to the detriment of the other. The employee probably will have a hard time negotiating away grounds for cause, because these clauses usually involve bad conduct for which the employee should be fired. Instead of negotiating the substance of reasonable and objective covenants, the employee instead should attempt to obtain reasonable cure periods and notice of violations. With those clauses in place, the practice must notify the employee of grounds for termination, and the employee will have a reasonable opportunity to correct such problems before being fired.

Most employment agreements also allow the parties to terminate "without cause" on 60 or 90 days' notice. Sometimes, based on the relative concerns of the practice or the employee OMS (for example, the practice is in a remote location, and it will take more time than usual to find a new OMS), the parties may desire to extend the duration of notice for "without cause" termination to 120 days or more.

Consequences of termination

The differences between the types of termination usually have significant financial consequences to the employee. Generally, if the employee terminates the employment without cause or the employer terminates with cause, the employee loses the right to receive unpaid bonuses. If the employer terminates the employment agreement without cause, the employee generally will have the right to receive bonus compensation at least through the date of termination or to have the bonus pro-rated based on performance through the date of termination. Occasionally, the employee also may be able to negotiate a severance package if he/she is fired without cause. This package should be the subject of early discussions and could be compelling if the associate has a good deal of negotiation leverage, is moving from a far distance, is leaving a profitable current employment situation, or is otherwise making a life-changing move to take the position. If the associate has little or no negotiation leverage, a severance package may not be warmly received by the practice.

Normally, if an employee owns shares or units in the practice, the practice will have a right to redeem, or repurchase, the shares or units. Generally, there is some penalty to the valuation of the redeemed shares/units if the employee is terminated for cause. Upon a termination for cause or resignation by the employee, the practice may be able to buy the shares/units back for the lesser of: (1) the price the employee paid for such shares/units; or (2) the fair market value of the shares/units (usually determined by a formula or appraisal). If the employee is fired without cause, the practice may be able to buy the shares/units back for the greater of (1) the price the employee paid for such shares/units; or (2) the fair market value of the shares/units. The financial differences between being fired with or without cause could be significant, and therefore the OMS should pay significant attention to the definition of "cause" and the time and ability to cure any grounds constituting cause.

Benefits and duties

The employment agreement must set forth the employee's benefits clearly and concisely. Language such as "Employee will receive benefits commensurate with other employee OMSs" should be avoided. This type of language, although common, does not really explain what benefits will be given to the employee. As mentioned elsewhere in this issue, the OMS can and should receive numerous benefits from the practice. Most of these benefits can be set forth quickly and clearly (eg, "The employee shall receive x days of vacation"). Other benefits may need more explanation and consideration in the employment agreement, but time should be taken to detail clearly these important parts of the relationship.

Ironically, the duties of the OMS employee often are given short shrift in the employment agreement; however, much like the benefits, the duties should be spelled out in detail so that expectations are established clearly. For example, junior physicians often complain that they are always on call. If the practice is honest about its call policies, and the employee is clear about those expectations, these complaints could be mitigated in the agreement by setting out how call is handled and how much call the employee OMS is expected to take.

Restrictive covenants

Most jurisdictions allow for practices to restrict their employee's postemployment activities through nonsolicitation of employees, nonsolicitation of customers, and noncompete covenants. The enforceability of these clauses varies from state to state, and in some states these clauses are unenforceable as a matter of public policy. It is essential that the OMS employee and practice seek competent legal counsel when drafting or reviewing these covenants.

Generally speaking, where noncompete clauses are permissible, they must be reasonable in geographic area, scope of the activity prohibited, and duration. The territory of a noncompete usually needs to be tied to the geographic area in which the OMS actually performed services for the practice. Noncompete clauses may be defined by radial miles from the practice(s) and/or by geographic areas such as counties or cities. For example, if an OMS performed services only in one of a practice's three locations, some states may require that the territory be tied only to area of the clientele of the one location where the OMS performed services, not to all of the practice's offices. Likewise, the scope of the activities prohibited usually must also be tied to the services the OMS actually performed for the practice. For example, some states may not allow an OMS to be restricted from performing general dentistry if the OMS performed only oral surgery for the practice. The duration of the restriction also must be a reasonable time frame for the practice to shore up its relationship with its clients. States differ greatly in how a reasonable duration is measured, and some prescribe it by statute, whereas others determine it on a case-by-case basis. The guidance of a lawyer knowledgeable in this area can help determine a reasonable duration for a noncompete clause in a particular state.

Nonsolicitation clauses prohibiting solicitation of a practice's employees or customers are not construed as strictly as noncompete clauses but still are sometimes difficult to enforce. Some jurisdictions will not enforce nonsolicitation clauses at all. Generally speaking, judges will follow a rule of reasonability in enforcing these clauses. Nonsolicitation clauses usually should be drafted to include a territory and a reasonable duration. Some states will enforce nonsolicitation clauses without a territory if the restriction on solicitation is limited to customers or employees with whom the employee had material contact during all or some recent part of the employee's employment with the practice. Additionally, states vary as to whether the nonsolicitation agreement may prevent a doctor from seeing patients he/she treated at a former practice or simply from soliciting such patients (ie, it may be permissible to see a patient if the patient seeks out that doctor rather than the doctor seeking out the former patient). Given the dramatic differences in rules and enforceability of noncompete and nonsolicitation clauses from state to state, it is imperative that a practice and OMS employee have lawyers well versed in this area review these restrictions.

Ownership of intellectual property

The understanding between the practice and the OMS with respect to ownership of intellectual property that the OMS may develop while an employee and the rights to use, transfer, license, sell, and exploit the intellectual property should be set forth clearly in the employment agreement. It is important for the OMS to understand that generally, as an employee, work or techniques created on company time or with company property will be owned by the practice. If the OMS is an entrepreneur or is academically minded and will be creating intellectual property, he/she should include language in the employment agreement to delineate clearly circumstances in which intellectual property is owned by the employee and not the practice. An example of such language is as follows:

> Employee shall own all inventions, ideas and work product that Employee develops entirely on Employee's own time without using the Practice's equipment, supplies, facilities, or trade secret information.

Confidentiality

Every company must protect its trade secrets and customer lists as valuable intellectual property. In addition, a medical practice also must protect sensitive patient information in a manner compliant with the Health Insurance Portability and Accountability Act of 1996, commonly referred to as "HIPAA." An OMS should expect to see rigorous confidentiality obligations in his/her employment agreement dealing both with information owned by the practice and private healthcare information of its patients. Usually the language that is presented with respect to HIPAA confidentiality is non-negotiable. An OMS, however, may consider certain exceptions to disclosure obligations with respect to confidential information that does not constitute health information of a patient. An example of exceptions to restrictions on use or disclosure is as follows:

> Notwithstanding anything contained to the contrary herein, the obligations imposed on Employee with respect to Confidential Information shall not apply to any Confidential Information which is not individual healthcare information or patient information *and*: (a) at the time of disclosure is generally available to the public or after the time of disclosure becomes generally available to the public through no act of the Employee; (b) was in the possession of the Employee prior to the disclosure and the receiving party can provide evidence to that fact; or (c) is made available to Employee by others who did not acquire such information, directly or indirectly, from the Practice and Employee can provide evidence of such.

Indemnification and insurance

Indemnification basically is a situation in which one party agrees to stand in the other's position to pay costs or damages that the other party may suffer. Usually a party will indemnify another only for acts or situations in which the party providing the indemnification can control events giving rise to the indemnity or in which, in all fairness, that party should be responsible for such costs and expenses. A company has liability for all of its employee's actions committed in the course of the employee's performance of services on behalf of the employer. The employment agreement for the OMS should indicate clearly that the OMS's acts and omissions (ie, malpractice) are covered by the practice's malpractice insurance while the OMS is employed by the practice. Typically, the OMS will be required to pay for and obtain tail insurance covering malpractice claims after the termination of the OMS from the practice's employment.

Buy-sell agreement, shareholder agreement, or operating agreement

The OMS and an established practice must weigh significant and numerous considerations when admitting a new OMS into the equity structure of an existing practice. Typically, the employment agreement will contain a provision with respect to the opportunity for an employee OMS to buy into the practice after a certain period of time and based on a certain set formula or valuation methodology. Once the mechanisms for the buy-in have been triggered, the practice usually will draft a series of documents for the current members or shareholders of the practice and the new OMS shareholder or member to sign. Depending on the size of the current practice, these documents may be fairly standard documents that many previous shareholders or members have signed (in the case of a large practice) or may be the first shareholders' agreement (in the case of a corporation) or operating agreement (in the case of a limited liability company) that has been drafted for the practice. If an OMS is buying into a large practice, the terms of the buy-in and the provisions surrounding ownership, dividends, buy-outs, and voting rights may be non-negotiable, or the OMS may have little flexibility in negotiating these terms. In such a situation the OMS should review the documents presented to him/her carefully and make sure that the documents accurately reflect the OMS's understanding of the deal. In addition, the OMS should determine whether this is the same deal others have received or if he/she is being treated differently. It is common for different treatment to be afforded to certain doctors within a practice, but the buying OMS needs to understand these differences before signing and paying his/her money into the practice.

More commonly, an OMS is buying into a small or mid-sized firm where there is some room for negotiation. Accordingly, the majority of this section discusses the provisions the OMS should look for in a shareholders' agreement or operating agreement. As an initial matter, the OMS should understand that it is bad form to use the negotiation of documents to change the general deal already reflected in the buy-in language of the employment agreement or the LOI. Usually, the negotiation of shareholders' agreements or an operating agreement deals strictly with legal language or issues that the parties have not discussed previously. Those issues usually are centered around: (1) buy-outs in the event of termination, retirement, death, or disability; (2) control and voting issues; (3) distributions; and (4) compensation and liability for the firm's debts and obligations.

Buy-outs

The OMS and the practice should specify how and when buy-outs of the shareholders or members can occur. Typically, a shareholder or member buy-out will occur when a shareholder or member is terminated as an employee, retires, becomes disabled, or dies. Usually, each of these circumstances is treated and valued differently.

As discussed previously, if the OMS is terminated for cause or resigns, his or her shares/units may be subjected to a lower valuation than if the OMS is terminated without cause. Generally, if the OMS is terminated with cause or resigns, the practice may have more favorable payment terms, such as payment of the purchase price under a promissory note over a 3- or 5-year period. The OMS should insist that if he/she is terminated without cause, his/her interest in the practice must be purchased for cash within a reasonable period after termination (30–90 days) and without discounts.

A practice also should buy out the interests of a member or shareholder when that member or shareholder dies. The members and practice should look into investing in insurance policies to cover the costs of such purchases. Insurance provides the members and practice an affordable means of obtaining the cash necessary to buy the units or shares without having to draw from personal or corporate funds. Knowing that insurance will pay the buy-out price also gives the members or shareholders comfort in knowing their estate will receive cash in exchange for their shares or membership interests.

For a practice with relatively few members or shareholders, the members or shareholders should look into cross-purchase arrangements in which the members or shareholders buy a deceased member or shareholder's interests in the practice with insurance proceeds. In this situation, each member takes an insurance policy on the life of the other member(s), the proceeds of which would purchase the other member's interests if such member dies. Such a purchase by one shareholder of another's is often referred to as a "cross-purchase." A cross-purchase using insurance proceeds allows the surviving member or shareholder to receive cash on a tax-free basis and also sets the member's tax basis in the shares purchased at the then-current purchase price.

Although a cross-purchase has tax benefits, this process begins to become unwieldy when a practice has three or more members or shareholders, because the number of required insurance policies grows exponentially. For instance, in a practice with two members or shareholders, each buys a policy on the other, requiring two policies. In a practice with three members or shareholders, each must buy a policy on the others, thereby requiring six policies for a cross-purchase. In such situations, the members or shareholders should look to forming an entity that is taxed as a partnership to hold the insurance policies on the lives of the members or shareholders. When a member or shareholder dies, the life insurance proceeds are distributed to the members or partners of the partnership-type entity holding the insurance policies without tax consequence. The members or shareholders then use those proceeds to purchase the shares of the deceased member or shareholder, thereby setting their tax basis in the purchased stock at the purchase price.

If the members or shareholders elect for the practice to repurchase their interests, the surviving members' or shareholders' interest in the practice will increase, but their tax basis in the interest in the company will not increase. Although such an arrangement may be more convenient and less costly on the front end, members or shareholders in a growing practice should consider spending money and time arranging a cross-purchase in the planning stages of a practice to gain the better long-term tax treatment of a cross-purchase buy-out.

A practice also should plan for the possibility of a member or shareholder becoming disabled. When a member or shareholder becomes disabled, the other members of the practice, rightly or wrongly, may feel that paying a share of the practice's profits to the nonworking member or shareholder is onerous. On the other hand, the disabled member or shareholder may need cash instead of the possibility of profits that accompany a membership or shareholder interest. Because of this possible scenario, a practice should have provisions dealing with the repurchase of a member's interest in the event of disability. Disability should be clearly defined and include only conditions for which a recovery is not likely for an extended period of time. Recovery periods from operations and longer illnesses for which recovery is likely should not trigger the buy-out.

The last type of common buy-out provisions have ominous names such as "Russian Roulette" or "Texas Shootout" but are essential if there is the potential for deadlock. These provisions typically allow one member or shareholder to make an offer to the other, setting the price at which the offering member is willing to buy or sell stock. The member or shareholder receiving the offer has the right to decide whether to take the price and sell his interests or to purchase the offering shareholder's or member's interest for the price stated. This system, by allowing one member to set the price and the other to choose whether to buy or sell at that price, is an inherently fair system that forces the member making the offer to come up with his/her best approximation of what fair market value would be for that interest, because that member must be willing either to buy or sell at that price.

Although this mechanism is inherently fair, it could favor a doctor who has more cash available. For instance, a doctor who has more cash available and sees the value of the practice rising in the near future could make an offer that, if cash needed to be paid right away, could force the other doctor to sell because of an inability to obtain funds to purchase the interest. To protect against this possible scenario, the OMS should insist that a provision be in place so that the member or shareholder receiving the offer can buy the interest of the member or shareholder making the offer over time with a promissory note to be secured by the shares or interest purchased. This provision levels the playing field, regardless of resources available to the doctors.

Control issues

In buying into a new practice, it is likely that the OMS will be buying a minority position. It therefore is important that the OMS attempt to obtain some customary protections so that he/she, as a minority shareholder or member, cannot be abused. Typically these provisions appear in a shareholders' agreement for practices operating as a corporation and in an operating agreement for practices operating as a limited liability company. A minority shareholder may have certain concerns that vary from practice to practice for which such minority owner would want prior consent. In general, a minority shareholder would want to obtain the right to consent before additional shares are issued to any current shareholder and possibly obtain rights of first refusal to those issuances if the majority refuses to allow a minority owner to have veto rights or review stock issuances. A minority owner also may attempt to obtain veto rights on the sale of the business, the business declaring bankruptcy, the dissolution of the practice, or the change in compensation among certain doctors. None of the foregoing options are always given; in fact, some are rarely given. If a minority shareholder needs to protect his/her investment in the practice, however, he/she should ask for some or all of these items.

Distributions

Typically, an OMS will be in a practice that is formed as either an S-corporation or an LLC. Distributions of S-corporation profits must be based on percentage of ownership, whereas distributions from an LLC may be structured in any number of ways. Minority owners of a corporation or LLC should make sure that their corporate documents discuss the timing of distributions. Members of an LLC also should review carefully how distributions will be made. Distributions in LLCs often are made first to members to the extent they have made loans to the LLC and then also may be distributed disproportionately among the members. A minority owner of an LLC must scrutinize the distributions section of an operating agreement because even though he/she might be a 10% owner of the company, this ownership position does not mean that he/she actually will receive 10% of the profits.

Liability for practice's liabilities

The newly admitted shareholder or member will want to make sure that he/she is not liable for the past indiscretions of the company. Debt obligations incurred by the practice before a new member or shareholder comes aboard may need to be segregated (as well as distributions before that member or shareholder is admitted). This matter should be delineated clearly in the shareholder agreement or the operating agreement so that all of the doctors understand who ultimately is responsible for certain debts and who ultimately is receiving distributions for certain periods of time.

Technology agreements

Technology has become a critical and an essential part of every medical practice, regardless of size or location. It is imperative that the OMS understand issues in technology agreements to purchase and deploy effectively technologies that will be useful and critical to the practice and the care of the practice's patients. There are many practice-management consulting firms that are extremely helpful to practices making purchases of hardware and software and that can provide good and sound referrals and advice in negotiating the business terms of technology acquisitions. When investing in technology, it is crucial that the OMS and his/her lawyer review carefully the terms of license agreements for software and ongoing maintenance and support agreements for technology purchased for his/her practice.

License agreements/Internet service provider agreements

Software solutions can be deployed locally on a practice's machines or over the Internet where data and the applications run remotely on a service provider's servers. These two types of technology deployment require different factors to be considered.

When acquiring software that will be deployed locally (ie, reside on the practice's hardware), the practice may benefit by keeping all of the sensitive patient data in-house and under the practice's control. The disadvantage is that the practice should have either consultants or in-house employees who can troubleshoot and effectively correct errors and downtime on the software and hardware located at the practice. A practice using a remotely located service provided by an application service provider benefits from not having to maintain competent, technologically savvy employees to minimize downtimes. The practice, however, could be sending sensitive client information protected under HIPAA. It therefore needs to demand rigorous confidentiality provisions with its service providers and to make sure that its service providers are HIPAA compliant. Typically, when acquiring a license to use software at the practice, the practice pays a one-time license fee along with ongoing maintenance and support fees. For an Internet-based service, a subscription fee, which includes the right to use the service, typically is charged on a monthly basis. Because the fees for the Internet service provider are spread out over time, this service typically is a more affordable short-term solution for a practice.

Regardless of whether a practice obtains a license to use software at its own facilities or uses an application service provider to fulfill its needs, the scope of the right to use the software (whether locally or through the Internet) must be examined carefully. Typical restrictions on rights to use include the number of seats, or authorized users, who can access the software and the number of transactions that can be processed in a given period of time. The OMS should ensure that the rights detailed in the licensing or service provider agreement are consistent with its understanding of what the OMS and his/her practice need.

It is not customary for software companies or providers to make representations or warranties with respect to performance. If a practice obtains services through an application service provider, however, it should insist on certain service level warranties, which usually are found in a service level agreement (SLA). SLAs usually contain uptime warranties that exceed 99% of the time. Other SLA warranties could be the retention, speed, and occasionally accuracy of certain calculations or processing of data.

It is important that the OMS review the SLAs carefully to make sure that critical functions are covered by the SLA and that appropriate damage amounts are set forth for breach of the SLA. The OMS also should consider allowing for termination of the agreement in the event of repeated breach of the SLAs. For instance, if the uptime SLA is breached for 2 consecutive months, this failure could be grounds for termination and a refund of any prepaid fees, together with any damage amounts related to the breach of the SLA. SLAs also are used in support and maintenance agreements for traditionally licensed software that resides locally at the practice. Software has errors and will break. Generally, code will be licensed in object code and therefore will be difficult, if not impossible, for a practice to fix. If an error occurs outside of the warranty period (generally a short period of time after a license is obtained), a practice will be able to have those errors fixed only if it has purchased support and maintenance from the licensor. Based on the type of software purchased, certain SLAs should be included in the support agreement. There should be differing response times based on the type of error that occurs. For instance, the response time should be much quicker for an error in a practice's billing software that causes it to not function at all than for an error causing a general annoyance that can be worked around or does not impact the functionality of the software. Typical response times for severe errors range from 1 to 4 hours with corrections for less severe errors being provided within a number of hours to a day or so, depending on the software.

Practices that purchase services over the Internet will obtain updates as the service provider puts the updates into production; however, practices that license software that resides locally on their hardware should insist in the support and maintenance agreement on receiving version updates and upgrades, which generally are made available to the licensor's customers who purchase maintenance. This provision will ensure that the practice receives up-to-date software advances and error corrections and bug fixes as they are made available.

For both the software and the application service provider models, a practice should attempt to receive warranties that the services provided or the software provided, as the case may be, do not infringe on anyone else's intellectual property rights and that they will not transmit viruses or other harmful code to the practice's software or the systems. The practice should be indemnified from any breach of these representations and warranties.

Technology agreements typically contain a limitation on liability section, which may or may not be enforceable, depending on the state in which the practice is located. Assuming that these provisions are enforceable, which they are in most states, a practice should scrutinize these limitations closely. Typically, the limitations prevent the practice from obtaining any consequential damages or lost profits caused by the software or the licensor's breach of the agreement. There are also usually caps on the licensor's liability that generally are tied to the amount of fees paid under the agreement or to the fees paid for a certain period of time under the agreement. The practice should attempt to modify these limitations on liability so that indemnification obligations and breaches of confidentiality are not limited in any form or fashion. It is imperative that breaches of confidentiality be excluded from the limitation on liability, because significant financial and reputational damage can occur to a practice if a patient's information is disclosed in an unauthorized fashion. Again, the practice should retain experienced counsel because significant aspects of the practice's day-to-day operations are impacted by technology agreements; if these agreements are not properly negotiated, the practice could be exposed to significant liabilities by failure to obtain certain remedies that typically are excluded in these agreements.

Most practices do not have a tremendous amount of negotiating power with technology providers or licensors. Therefore, it is important that the practice pick its battles when negotiating these agreements and, most importantly, that it does its due diligence on these firms before entering into any contract. Medical practice consultants can be an invaluable resource in providing referrals, as can other doctors who use the service or software. Well-negotiated agreements can be good protection when things go bad, but it is much better to be assured through due diligence activities that the likelihood of bad things happening is low.

Summary

The OMS will deal with various, complex contracts, starting from the moment he/she begins negotiating with his/her first private practice employer until the time he/she buys into a practice and then makes decisions on the practice's purchases and business decisions. A sound knowledge of typical considerations and customary terms will be essential for the OMS throughout his/her career. This article only touches on the agreements and considerations commonly faced by an OMS and considers only the major issues in those agreements. Legal counsel will be needed to negotiate many of these agreements; however, the OMS should have a sound background in the general terms and common conditions discussed in this article.

Credentialing and Privileging for the Oral and Maxillofacial Surgeon

Steven R. Nelson, DDS, MS

Rocky Mountain Oral and Maxillofacial Surgery, 6850 East Hampden Avenue, Denver, CO 80224, USA

The Centers for Medicare and Medicaid Services (CMS) have established quality and patient safety requirements called conditions of participation (COPs) that hospitals must fulfill to be eligible for Medicare payment. To show compliance, hospitals and ambulatory surgery centers can be accredited by an authorized body, such as the Joint Commission on Accreditation of Healthcare Organizations (Joint Commission), American Osteopathic Association (AOA), or Accreditation Association for Ambulatory Health Care, Inc. (AAAHC), or reviewed by a state certification agency under contract to the CMS [1]. Currently, 82% of Medicare-eligible hospitals are accredited by the Joint Commission [2]. In addition to establishing COP compliance, organizations proclaim accreditation to be a measure of professional achievement and provision of quality health care [2,3]. Accreditation standards have been developed to promote continuous compliance with quality and safety requirements. Integral to these requirements are the specific standards for the credentialing and privileging of medical staff members.

For many physicians, the mentioning of the terms "credentialing" and "privileging" can bring a feeling of angst. The initial application for medical staff membership and clinical privileging or the application requesting new privileges can be an intimidating task. Determining the competency of practitioners to provide high-quality and safe patient care is one of the most important decisions that accredited health care organizations must make. These organizations must provide a fair and credible process to credential and privilege

their members, which requires significant data collection and evaluation [4,5]. Whether the oral and maxillofacial surgeon (OMS) is applying for initial appointment to a medical staff or for reappointment, two steps must be completed: (1) credentials must be verified, and (2) appropriate privileges must be approved [5,6]. Understanding the terms involved in the processes allows the OMS to prepare better for and gain his or her requested membership and privileges.

Credentialing is the process of obtaining, verifying, and assessing the qualifications of the OMS to provide services in or for an organization. These qualifications include the OMS's education, training, and experience. Privileging is the process whereby a specific scope and content of clinical privileges are authorized for an OMS by an organization based on evaluation of the individual's credentials and performance. This performance can be based on demonstrated competence and judgment.

Currently, hospitals and ambulatory surgery centers are the most common organizations that credential and authorize clinical privileges for the OMS. Credentialing is also performed by additional organizations, such as health maintenance organizations and other third-party health insurance carriers. Recently, states are beginning to perform a standardized credentialing service.

Qualifications of the oral and maxillofacial surgeon

Oral and maxillofacial surgery is defined by the American Dental Association (ADA) and the American Association of Oral and Maxillofacial Surgeons (AAOMS) as the specialty of dentistry that includes the diagnosis, surgical, and

E-mail address: snelson@rmoms.com

adjunctive treatment of diseases, injuries, and defects involving the functional and esthetic aspects of the bone and soft tissues of the oral and maxillofacial region. As a recognized specialty of dentistry, it is regulated by state dental boards.

The oral and maxillofacial surgeon is a uniquely qualified member of any medical staff based on education, training, and patient services provided. In response to patients' needs and requests, in combination with scientific and technologic advancements, the scope of practice for oral and maxillofacial surgery has evolved into a surgical specialty with multiple areas of interest. Many surgical procedures are performed in a hospital or outpatient surgical center based on their complexity or need for additional health care team support. To provide care at these organizations, practitioners must obtain appropriate privileges. The medical staff office of most major hospitals and ambulatory surgery centers is familiar with the extensive training of the OMS. In some cases, however, there still exists the need to educate individuals or committees about the education, training, and experience of the OMS.

The education of the OMS ensues after graduation from dental school, having earned a doctor of dental surgery (DDS) or doctor of dental medicine (DMD) degree. The OMS completes a hospital-based oral and maxillofacial surgical residency accredited by the ADA Commission on Dental Accreditation (CODA), a nationally recognized accrediting body that is approved by the US Department of Education. The residency spans a minimum of 48 months of full-time training, as required in the accreditation Standards for Advanced Specialty Education Programs in Oral and Maxillofacial Surgery [7]. On successful completion, the resident is competent in patient assessment, anesthesia, dentoalveolar surgery, facial trauma surgery, maxillofacial pathology, maxillofacial reconstructive surgery, orthognathic surgery, cleft and craniofacial surgery, temporomandibular joint surgery, and facial cosmetic surgery. Residents spend at least 30 months devoted to clinical oral and maxillofacial surgery and at least 12 months assigned to the hospital anesthesia, medical, and surgical services. An essential component of the residency training is development of competency for all residents to take a complete medical history and perform a comprehensive physical evaluation [7]. Some residency programs offer additional educational opportunity for the OMS to earn a doctor of medicine (MD) degree. It needs to be emphasized that the training in oral and maxillofacial surgery is the same for the single-degreed (dental degree only) or dual-degreed (dental and medical degrees) OMS.

Credentialing and privileging process

Individual hospitals have their own protocol for credentialing and privileging medical staff members. The following outline should give the reader a good understanding of the complexity and time commitment required by the applicant and medical staff office and committees.

Preapplication

After a request for application for appointment to the medical staff, an application request form is forwarded to the applicant. Individuals must be able to demonstrate (1) that they are an MD, DDS, or DMD, with a valid license in good standing to practice in their state; (2) that they have obtained and maintain professional liability insurance in accordance with the hospital, state, or federal law; and (3) that they have successfully completed an approved residency program. On receipt of a completed application request form, the hospital chief executive officer (CEO) or appropriate designee verifies the contents. If the initial requirements are met, the CEO provides a response to the requesting practitioner, which may or my not include an application. If the requirements are not met, the potential applicant should request an opportunity for an informal discussion with the president of the medical staff and CEO to help make his or her case for appointment.

Application for initial appointment

Application for staff appointment is then submitted by the applicant. Most applications include a completed application form with current photo identification, a request for clinical privileges, a copy of the applicant's current license and Drug Enforcement Agency (DEA) certification, a copy of the applicant's current professional liability insurance policy, copies of certificates and letters confirming completion of an approved residency/training program or other educational curriculum, a copy of certificate or letter from appropriate specialty board regarding board status, and letters of recommendation from persons who have recently worked with the applicant and directly observed his or her professional performance, which are usually sent directly to the CEO or medical staff office [5].

The applicant should have access to the hospital and medical staff bylaws, policies, procedures, rules, regulations, manuals, guidelines, and requirements. It is imperative to obtain, read, and understand these documents before submitting the application. In submitting a signed application, the applicant may be authorizing the hospital representatives to (1) consult with persons who can provide information about his or her competence and qualifications; (2) inspect records pertaining to professional qualification, physical and mental health status, and his or her professional and ethical qualifications; and (3) provide information about the applicant to other hospitals, medical associations, and licensing boards. In addition, the applicant releases from liability the hospital and individuals and organizations providing information. The applicant further agrees to provide and update information requested on the original application and subsequent reapplications for reappointment and privilege request forms or of any change in information provided on the most current application form [5]. Most hospital bylaws maintain provisions for automatic withdrawal of an application for any misrepresentation, misstatement, or omission from the application. In addition, a protocol for applicants previously denied membership should be available.

Processing the application

Once an application has been received in the medical staff office, it is reviewed for completeness. If additional information is required, there is usually a strict time frame in which to provide or reply to the requested material. If an applicant does not respond within the time frame, many hospitals consider the application withdrawn. Know your hospital bylaws. For a practitioner who has an initial application deemed withdrawn, he or she may not be entitled to procedural rights that protect practitioners already on staff or applicants who have a complete application.

On receipt of a completed application, the CEO verifies its contents and collects additional information, such as securing clinical reference questionnaires and administrative references from past practice settings, verification of the applicant's clinical work during the past 12 to 24 months, information from the National Practitioners' Data Bank (NPDB), information from state dental and medical boards, verification of licensure status in all current or past states of licensure, information from the American Medical Association (AMA) Physician Masterfile Profile if applicable, and documentation of compliance with the hospital tuberculosis (TB) testing policy [5,8].

When all information has been obtained and verified, the completed application is forwarded to the appropriate department chairman for review and report by that department. The department chair may solicit additional information regarding the applicant and may request an interview with the applicant. Once the department has completed its review of the application, the department chair makes a report to the credentials committee. The completed application with the department report is then reviewed by the credentials committee. The credentials committee may request additional information and/or an interview with the applicant. The credentials committee reports to the medical executive committee (MEC). The department and credentials committee report addresses the applicant's eligibility, education, training, qualifications, and experience for medical staff appointment and clinical privileges requested. The MEC reviews all these reports, the application, and all supporting and additional information. The MEC may request additional information and/or an interview with the applicant. The MEC forwards to the hospital board of trustees (usually through the CEO) a recommendation as to the granting of staff appointment, staff category, department affiliation, and clinical privileges and any special conditions regarding appointment. If the recommendation is adverse, the MEC usually contacts the applicant before presenting the recommendation to the board until the applicant has exhausted or waived his or her procedural rights as outlined in the hospital and medical staff bylaws.

Governing body/board of trustees action

The board of trustees may adopt or reject in whole or in part a favorable recommendation from the MEC or defer the recommendation back to the credentials committee for further consideration. Favorable action by the board is effective as its final action. If the board's action is adverse, an avenue for appeals utilizing due process and the inclusion of fair hearings must be available to the applicant.

The notice of final decision by the board is given to the CEO, MEC, and chairman of each applicable department. The decision and notice should include staff category to which the applicant is appointed, the department to which he or she is assigned, the clinical privileges he or she may exercise, and any special conditions attached to the appointment.

Most hospitals have strict time frames for this process. Even in expedited proceedings, this process is time-consuming. The applicant needs to be prepared, understand the time frame involved, and know the information he or she needs to provide. The process is the same for the senior resident approaching completion of his or her program as for the established practitioner who is joining a new medical staff.

Preparing for the credentialing and privileging process

Before making an application for initial appointment on a hospital medical staff, the OMS should address the following concerns.

Know your state's dental practice law

Obtain a copy of the current state dental practice law by contacting the state board of dental examiners. Specifically, the applicant should know his or her state's (1) definitions of dentistry and oral and maxillofacial surgery, (2) position on recognizing oral and maxillofacial surgery as a specialty, (3) defined scope of the oral and maxillofacial surgery practice, and (4) existing statutes that pertain to the practice of oral and maxillofacial surgery or specific surgical privileges desired. If your state does not have contemporary definitions of dentistry or oral and maxillofacial surgery or has a limited scope of practice defined, collaboration with your states OMS society and state dental association is recommended to modify the state dental practice law. The AAOMS can provide excellent resources for this labor-intensive endeavor.

Know the hospital for which you are seeking appointment

Applicants should learn the hospital's medical staff structure. Know the department to which you would be appointed. You should ascertain whether there is a specific dental or oral and maxillofacial department or if oral and maxillofacial surgery is a part of the surgery department. Know how many OMSs are on staff and their category of appointment and activity level in the hospital. If there are few OMSs with minimal activity, the medical staff may require more information regarding your training and competence. Learn who is on the MEC and credentials committee. If possible, make an effort to meet these individuals to show your interest in the hospital and commitment to the hospital mission. Ascertain the level of commitment to patients undergoing oral and maxillofacial surgery, including equipment needed for your scope of practice. Obtain and learn the bylaws and rules and regulation of the hospital and medical staff and the mission and vision of the hospital. Understand the hospital's credentialing and privileging protocol, including the appeal process. It is important to understand the medical staff political structure at the time of your application. As officers and committee members change, so does the political nature, and choosing when to add a new privilege may depend on who is on the MEC and credentials committee and who is the chair of the department. Obviously, members who are knowledgeable about oral and maxillofacial surgery training, education, and experience can make the process run smoothly. Less informed members may require education. Unfortunately, a member of any of these committees who is hostile to the scope of oral and maxillofacial surgery practice can make the entire process challenging.

Know the Joint Commission (or the accrediting body of your hospital) medical staff standards

A working knowledge of these standards can be helpful during dialog with the medical staff office and members of the MEC or credentials committee. In 2007, the Joint Commission introduced three new concepts to the credentialing and privileging standards. The three concepts are (1) General Competencies, which integrated the six areas of general competency that were developed by the Accreditation Council for Graduate Medical Education and the American Board of Medical Specialties; (2) Focused Professional Practice Evaluation, designed to evaluate a specific aspect of a practitioner's performance; and (3) Ongoing Professional Practice Evaluation, which is designed to continuously evaluate a practitioner's performance and establish a more efficient evidence-based privilege renewal process [5]. Current standards require verification of current licensure at the granting of initial privileges, at the granting of reprivileging, and at the time of license expiration. Verification of the applicant's education and training should be obtained from the original source of the specific credential. According to the most recent hospital standards, primary sources include the certifying boards approved by the ADA, letters from professional schools, and letters from residency programs for completion of training [5]. The standards for privileging include criteria to grant or deny privileges or to renew an existing privilege. These must be objective and evidence based. Each of the criteria used must be consistently applied for all practitioners holding that privilege [4,5,9,10]. Contact the hospital's accrediting body for the most current accreditation standards. Pay particular attention to the section or chapter on medical staff.

Assemble required documentation

Read the application thoroughly to identify all required information. Verification of state licensure, malpractice insurance, Basic Life Support (BLS)/Advanced Cardiac Life Support (ACLS) training, TB test result, and continuing medical and dental education is required, as is your National Provider Identifier (NPI) number and taxonomy code. In addition, you need to document the types and number of procedures you performed in the past 2 years, be prepared to document and defend any reports to the NPDB, and obtain a letter from the director your training program or chair of the department where you previously were privileged.

Request appropriate privileges

As with all practitioners, the granting of clinical privileges should be based on education, training, experience, and demonstrated competence and judgment [4,5,8–11].

Hospitals may utilize core privileging or procedure list privileging or some combination. Core privileging provides a generalized or specific list of the classic scope of practice for oral and maxillofacial surgery, including history and physical examination (H&P) privileges. Core privileges are approved as a block of privileges unless otherwise specified. Usually, additional privileges can be requested that require further documentation of training and competence. Hospitals that privilege by procedure provide an exhaustive list of procedures and request the number performed of each in the past 2 years to obtain or maintain privileges for that procedure. In either case, if you are requesting privileges for head and neck surgery, cosmetic surgery, laser surgery, and liposuction, be prepared to document your education, training, and experience.

Additional criteria as established by the hospital and medical staff need to be met. Documentation of completion of an approved residency training program in oral and maxillofacial surgery, documentation of performance of the procedure, and certification by the American Board of Oral and Maxillofacial Surgery (ABOMS) are common criteria. The CMS have clearly stated that it is not acceptable to utilize board certification as the only criterion in granting privileges. For initial or new privileging, case observations may be required. It is paramount that the institution has an established and clear privileging process that is applied uniformly and fairly for all practitioners. It is also important to know that privileges may cross departments and that no one department can lay claim to a particular privilege.

Special privileging circumstances

Request for new privileges

This depends on several variables, which include the following:

- How the hospital delineates privileges (ie, core versus procedure list)
- If you have participated in additional education and possess a new skill for a privilege previously not requested
- If this is a new procedure or emerging technology previously not privileged at the hospital

You should be ready to support your new privilege request by providing the educational courses taken, a letter from a person who has personal knowledge of your ability regarding the new privilege, a list documenting your performance of said privilege, and a radiographic/photographic/narrative before and after documentation. For privileging in new procedures and emerging technologies, you must document additional training in this new scope of practice [12]. You should also verify and document that your malpractice carrier covers this new scope.

Denial of privileges

If a practitioner has a requested privilege denied, the hospital appeal process should be followed. It is important to make sure that the hospital and medical staff followed their own rules, as outlined in the bylaws, during the privileging process. Support to appeal the process may be obtained through study of the hospital accrediting body standards, study of the hospital and medical staff bylaws, and AAOMS.

As stated previously, and this can not be stressed enough, the granting of privileges should be based uniformly on education, training, experience, and demonstrated competence and judgment. If the privilege requested was denied despite appropriate training, education, and competency, you may need to seek outside counsel to challenge the decision.

Revocation of privileges

When a hospital becomes aware of health care quality concerns regarding a medical staff member, investigation of this concern should be carried out in accordance with the hospital and medical staff bylaws. If the concern is verified, necessary actions are taken, which may include limitation, suspension, revocation, or nonrenewal of staff privileges [13]. This can be devastating to a practitioner and his or her practice and may be reportable to the NPDB. The practitioner may also be required to notify his or her medical malpractice carrier of this action. The hospital bylaws outline an appeals process for you to follow. Because of the myriad of existing legal theories and depending on jurisdiction, an OMS who has had an adverse action taken against his or her privileges should consult with legal counsel [4,6,13–15].

Current challenges to credentialing and privileging

The AAOMS Division of Advanced Education and Professional Affairs monitors inquiries regarding the credentialing and privileging of the OMS. During the time frame from 2001 to 2006, the areas that generated the most inquiries were H&P privileges (86 inquiries), full-scope practice (65 inquiries), development of core privileging (61 inquiries), equitable trauma/emergency room call (45 inquiries), and cosmetic privilege (39 inquiries) [16]. To address these concerns, the AAOMS Committee on Hospital and Interprofessional Affairs has developed a core privilege document to support OMS full-scope privileges based on CODA residency standards and the AAOMS parameters of care. In addition, guidelines for credentialing in facial cosmetic surgery have been developed. You can obtain these guidelines by contacting the AAOMS [17].

It is surprising that the performance of the H&P by OMSs continues to generate the most inquiries [14,16,18]. An essential component of an accredited oral and maxillofacial surgery residency program is educating residents to take a complete medical history and perform a comprehensive physical evaluation. Since 1981, the Joint Commission has recognized the competency of the OMS to perform the H&P for admission to a hospital facility [18]. According to the Joint Commission, the current definition of an OMS is "An individual who has successfully completed a postgraduate program in oral and maxillofacial surgery accredited by a nationally recognized accrediting body approved by the US Department of Education. As determined by the medical staff, the individual is also currently competent to perform a complete history and physical examination in order to assess the medical, surgical, and anesthetic risks for the proposed operative and other procedure(s)" [5].

The CMS provides even stronger support for the OMS to perform the H&P, defining it as a condition of participation found in section 482.22 (Condition of Participation: Medical staff). This was recently reconfirmed in the November 2006 *Federal Register* through discussion of the time frame completion of the H&P. Specifically, section 482.22(c)(5) states: "This requirement expands the timeframe for completion of the history and physical examination... A physician (as defined in section 1861 (r) of the Act), oromaxillofacial surgeon, or other qualified individual could complete the history and physical examination in accordance with State law and hospital policy..." The act further pointed out that "For clarification in this final rule, the specific reference to oromaxillofacial surgeons has been retained. However, based on hospital policy and State law, the pool of 'other qualified individual' can be restricted" [19].

The granting of all clinical privileges must be an objective evidenced-based process and free from turf battles. As previously stated, criteria utilized in granting privileges must be consistently applied to all practitioners holding that privilege. Again, it cannot be stressed enough that clinical privileges granted to all practitioners should be based on education, training, experience, and demonstrated competence and judgment. These tenets are supported by the Joint Commission, ADA, AAOMS, AMA, and CMS [5,8–11,19].

Summary

The practice of oral and maxillofacial surgery is constantly changing. This change not only includes an increased scope of practice but modifications in the settings where the oral and maxillofacial surgeon provides these services. OMSs play an essential role in the delivery of comprehensive health care in the hospital setting. Unfortunately, there seems to be a trend that many OMSs are not joining hospital medical staffs. Clearly, most of the procedures that OMSs perform are on an outpatient basis and office based. For the significantly medically compromised patient, for the patient undergoing major orthognathic and reconstruction, and for many patients with trauma, however, their care is best performed in a hospital setting. Obtaining and maintaining hospital staff membership is in our patients' best interest. You now know that the credentialing and privileging process is a labor-intensive and time-consuming endeavor but one that is necessary. Your preparation and knowledge of the process, hospital bylaws, rules and regulations, and accreditation standards is essential. Your initial well-informed and collaborative approach with the medical staff office and members of the credentialing and privileging committees is likely to be invaluable and can help to ensure an effective, fair, and efficient process.

Appendix A

Credentialing and Privileging Resources

American Association of Oral and Maxillofacial Surgeons, Division of Advanced Education and Professional Affairs, 9700 West Bryn Mawr Avenue, Rosemont, IL 60018, 800-822-6637; available at: www.aaoms.org.

American Dental Association, Council on Access, Prevention, and Interprofessional Relations, 211 East Chicago Avenue, Chicago, IL 60611, 800-621-8099; available at: www.ada.org.

Joint Commission on Accreditation of Healthcare Organizations, One Renaissance Boulevard, Oakbrook, Terrace, IL 60181, 630-792-5000; Central Office, 630-792-5900; Standards questions, available at: www.jointcommission.org.

Commission on Dental Accreditation, 211 East Chicago Avenue, Chicago, IL 60611, 312-440-4653; available at: www.ada.org.

Centers for Medicare and Medicaid Services; available at: www.cms.hhs.gov.

American Osteopathic Association, 142 East Ontario Street, Chicago, IL 60611, 800-621-1773; available at: www.do-online.org.

Accreditation Association for Ambulatory Health Care, 5250 Old Orchard Road, Suite 200, Skokie, IL 60077, 847-853-6060; available at: www.aaahc.org.

References

[1] Sprague L. Hospital oversight in Medicare: accreditation and deeming authority. Washington DC: National Health Policy Forum; NHPF Issue Brief. No. 802, 2005. p. 1–15.

[2] Government Accountability Office (GAO). CMS needs additional authority to adequately oversee patient safety in hospitals. Washington DC: GAO; 2004. p. 04–850.

[3] Chyna JT. Improving privileging and credentialing. Go beyond the minimum standards with best practices. Healthc Exec 2005;20(4):50–1.

[4] Hirsch EA. Fighting hospital privileges. Fam Pract Manag 2004;11(3):69–74.

[5] Joint Commission on Accreditation of Healthcare Organizations. Comprehensive accreditation manual for hospitals. Oakbrook Terrace (IL): Joint Commission Resources, Inc; 2007.

[6] Curtis T, Russell LA. Challenges in medical staff credentialing. Med Staff Couns 1993;7(4):23–9.

[7] Commission on Dental Accreditation. Standards for advanced specialty education programs in oral and maxillofacial surgery. Chicago: CODA; 2006. p. 1–34.

[8] AAOMS guidelines to hospital and ambulatory credentialing in OMS procedures. Rosemont (IL): American Association of Oral and Maxillofacial Surgeons; 2006. p. 1–5.

[9] American Dental Association Council on Access, Prevention and Interprofessional Relations. Guidelines for the delineation of clinical privileges in dentistry. Chicago (IL): 1995. p. 1–3.

[10] American Medical Association Policy H-230.972. Physician credentialing and privileging. 2005. Available at: www.ama-assn.org.

[11] Joint Commission on Accreditation of Health Care Organizations and the American Dental Association. Guide to joint commission hospital accreditation resources for dentists, Oakbrook Terrace (IL): 1998.

[12] Sachdeve AK, Russell TR. Safe introduction of new procedures and emerging technologies in surgery: education, credentialing, and privileging. Surg Oncol Clin N Am 2007;16:101–14.

[13] Dallon CW. Understanding judicial review of hospitals' physician credentialing and peer review decisions. Temple Law Rev 2000;73:597–679.

[14] Donlon WC. Regulatory aspects of hospital credentialing. In: Smith RE, editor. Oral and maxillofacial surgery clinics of North America. Philadelphia: WB Saunders; 1995. p. 691–702.

[15] Cultice PN. Privileging: physicians are protected by the Americans with Disabilities Act. J Health Hosp Law 1995;28(3):163–72, 192.

[16] AAOMS Committee on Hospital and Interprofessional Affairs. Comparative logs 2001–2006 and trends. Rosemont (IL): 2007.
[17] Available at: www.aaoms.org.
[18] Donlon WC. Credentialing and privileging for oral and maxillofacial surgeons. In: Fonseca RJ, editor. Oral and maxillofacial surgery, vol. 1. Philadelphia: WB Saunders; 2000. p. 520–30.
[19] Medicare and Medicaid programs; hospital conditions of participation final rule. Fed Regist 2006; vol. 71: 42 CFR Part 482, no. 227, Monday November 27, 6869.

The Modern Oral and Maxillofacial Surgery Office
W. Scott Jenkins, DMD, MD

Jenkins & Morrow Oral and Maxillofacial Surgery, 216 Fountain Court, Suite 110A, Lexington, KY 40509, USA

The specialty of oral and maxillofacial surgery (OMS) today offers the surgeon the ability to practice a diverse scope of practice depending on the individual's preference and training. Facial cosmetic, head and neck oncologic, craniofacial, and traditional oral and maxillofacial and implant surgery at varying intensities can be pursued in one's practice. The diversity among surgeons in the specialty is not limited to a set of surgical skills but is also seen in regard to practice design and patient care philosophies.

This article discusses the modern OMS practice and those elements that are critical to developing a practice in today's atmosphere of technologic advancement as it relates to patient care and satisfaction. Although there are many aspects of developing a new practice, the following discussion focuses on the elements that facilitate modern patient care and office operation.

The most crucial aspect of designing a new practice or revamping an existing practice is keeping in mind that the outward appearance of the practice is the first impression of the type of care patients will receive when entering the facility. As a result, the surgeon should attempt to design a space that facilitates easy patient accessibility with ergonomics for patient flow, staff use, and care delivery. By paying attention to this plan, sound patient care and a unique facility can become one of the greatest marketing tools the contemporary oral and maxillofacial surgeon has in the current competitive market.

Design concepts

The overall design goals for an office are to create an environment that is comfortable and stress-free along with making a first impression that is representative of the practice's quality of care. The state-of-the art office could be reflected in the colors, materials, and level of design incorporating a distinctive look not typical of a dental or medical practice.

The emphasis on focal points enables patients to quickly feel comfortable. For example, features such as a water wall etched with signage allows the patients to identify the office suite and enjoy a soothing waterfall as they spend time in the reception/waiting area (Fig. 1). The sound and action of the falling water evokes a sense of calmness.

A reception desk, the first impression, may incorporate striking architectural shapes with a combination of forms and materials to create a strong focal point (Fig. 2). There may be colors on custom casework that introduce the color palette for the entire office using the comfort of rich colors and warm neutrals. The contrast of light and dark woods can create a balance and harmony in wood tones.

Oversize seating in the waiting area enables patients to be comfortable as they come in, sit down, and relax. Nontraditional settees can bring an element of distinction to the overall feel of the space. Art throughout the office provides interest and additional focal points for patients as they move through the space (Fig. 3). Colors and textures reflect the palette introduced in other focal points maintaining a common theme throughout.

Office floor plan

Picture yourself as a patient or patient's parent walking into the local oral and maxillofacial surgeon's office for the first time. After parking, you walk into the waiting room to register because you tried online but there was no website for registration or directions. You walk into the

E-mail address: jenxdmdmd@yahoo.com

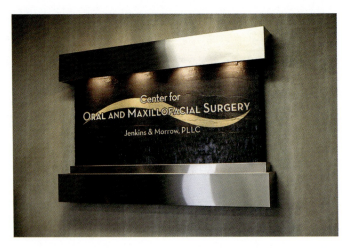

Fig. 1. Combination water feature and signage used to create interest and identification of the practice with a relaxing attribute when added to the lobby.

waiting room and you look around. Entering through the door there is a television on a makeshift stand with the cable line taped to the floor next to the baseboard. The local news in on and the picture is fuzzy at best. The walls are white with few or no pictures and there are fluorescent lights in the ceiling. At your feet is medical-grade ocean-blue carpet circa 1970. There is a glass enclosure behind which the receptionist sits; it is hard to hear the receptionist through the circular port and over the sound of a nitrogen-powered handpiece only 8 ft away. You are handed a stack of paperwork to fill out and asked to return to the window when you are finished and the staff will get you right back to a room.

Now picture the same scenario only this time you enter having had the directions printed from the practice's well-designed and easily navigated Web site. While on the Web site you were offered the opportunity to register so you have already given your insurance and demographic information. You enter through the door and there is a rich hardwood entry that is well-lighted, inviting you to the reception desk that is well-decorated in rich colors. There is colorful artwork on the wall and a flat screen monitor, which is displaying high-resolution, informative patient information in one corner and national news in another. You give the staff your name and they report they are ready to seat you in your room if you are ready.

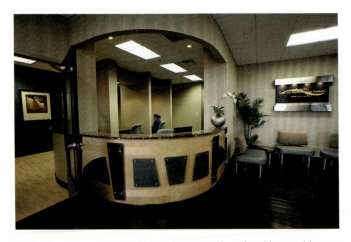

Fig. 2. Reception area with geometric case work and architectural interest.

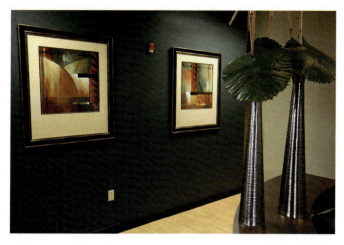

Fig. 3. Examples of artwork that bring in a warm color palette and help coordinate design elements.

The impressions generated from these scenarios are quite different. Although the care delivered may be the same at both offices, the latter allows the facility to market not only the care but also the atmosphere established based on the good first impression.

In today's competitive market the OMS office must be able to not only support the clinical responsibility of patient care but also incorporate design elements that esthetically help set the tone for future patient care. These design elements include proper color selection, lighting, furniture, and artwork, which together allow your office to initiate the marketing plan. A poorly furnished and decorated office may send the message indirectly that the level of care may be less than superior. The design and coordination of the waiting area and the entire office should be done in consultation with a trusted design professional, preferably someone who has a proven track record in dental and medical offices. This consultation allows for desirable furnishings that will stand up to the rigors of the office.

The basic office layout or floor plan is important for many reasons. The flexibility of the floor plans often relates to the space in which the office must be constructed. The ideal scenario allows for the desired office space to be oriented on a piece of property that offers ease of access and good visibility to the public. This ideal is usually not the case, however; the space is acquired and the layout design is based on the pre-existing exterior wall design.

The organization of the office is crucial to the practice's ease of use of the facility. Having the proper layout increases productivity, decreases staff frustration, and decreases stress on the surgeon and patients. The basic concept is to design the office so that three different zones exist: the clinical zone, the public zone, and the staff zone [1,2]. The basic tenet is to keep treatment and patient care in the clinical zone away from the public zone that is reserved for the waiting room and business area. The staff zone offers areas for staff to retreat, use the bathroom, eat, or break, and is away from the clinical and public zones.

When initially designing an office or remodeling an existing one these zoning principles should be applied (Fig. 4). Working with a trained medical or dental architect helps ease this process and allows the patient to transition through the practice in a streamlined manner. The aspects of office size, number of rooms per surgeon, and size of rooms should be reviewed with a trained architect but also rely heavily on budget, office rough size, and personal preference. The basic ergonomics of each space depend on the tasks performed in that space. For example, in the clinical zone (operatories), the cabinet layout depends on whether the surgeon is right or left handed, sits or stands, wears a head light, or uses ceiling mounted light sources. Based on these elements the proper design may be selected. This consideration is also true for staff areas and computer monitor heights, keyboard orientation, and phone outlets.

An important area not to overlook within the clinical zone is the sterilization area. This space is a regulator to patient flow. If instruments cannot be turned over then patient care is slowed or halted. This area should be of sufficient size to

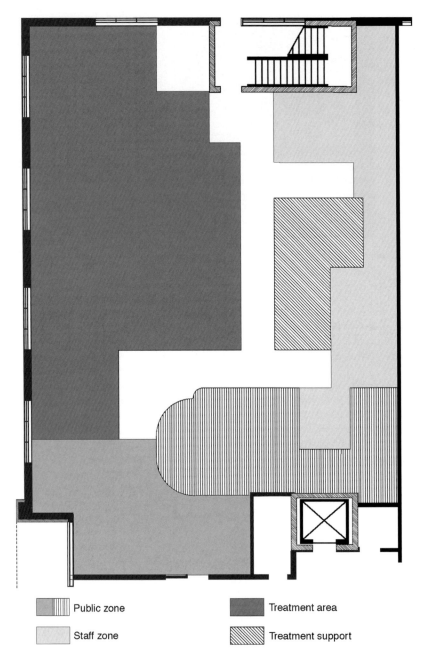

Fig. 4. Area floor plan before final design that establishes designated spaces and coordinates flow.

accommodate the number of treatment rooms, usually requiring 3 to 3.5 ft per operatory for up to eight operatories [2]. These areas should be centrally located within the clinical zone and designed so contaminated instruments can be managed in a designated area, processed (sterilized), and placed in the designated clean area. This concept was developed by the Centers for Disease Control and further delineated guidelines can be found online. Today there are various instrument container systems or cassettes and instrument washing devices that can help manage these instruments in larger quantities with an overall decrease in handling and processing time. A full detailed description of the ideal sterilization room and the available equipment is beyond the scope of this article but these basic principles should be in place.

Spending the appropriate time in planning the office layout in the long run allows the contemporary OMS office to be productive and to facilitate seamless patient care (Fig. 5). Once the layout is determined and the office consistently appeals to the patient's eye, the practice itself becomes an extension of the type of care the patients perceive they will receive.

Digital operating systems

Although computer software packages for the management of dental and medical practices are certainly not new there are several highly specific options on the market today for oral and maxillofacial surgeons. Choosing from these, which include OMS Vision by Discus Dental, WinOMS CS by Practice Works, Oral Surgery-Exec by DSN Software Inc., and Windent OMS by Windent Practice Management Solutions, should be based on personal preference. This personal preference should be related to the characteristic features for the software setup and how they relate to ease of use for you and your staff, cost, 24-hour real-time technical support, number of upgrades per year, customization, and capability for integration with future and current technologies, such as wireless pads, digital radiology, remote use, and hand-held personal digital assistants (PDAs). Each of these systems can be reviewed in detail on the Web and area representatives can arrange for on-site introduction with navigation of the systems to highlight each one's capabilities.

The contemporary OMS practice is one that is digital throughout and allows the surgeon, staff, and patients to acquire, input, and process needed information effectively based on the hardware and software design. This ability requires coordination with the office floor plan and projected needs of the staff and surgeon to appropriately locate and disperse the selected hardware. Once the number and position of all work stations is determined the appropriate management software must be chosen. The ideal software package allows the clinical staff and surgeon efficient use of the patient record for charting, image visualization, health alerts, and documentation. Similarly for the clerical or billing staff, ease of data entry, scheduling, billing, electronic claim submissions, and statement generation should be optimized. Finally, the software must allow generation of reports and practice analyses that have tangible meaning to the business (eg, production versus collection analysis, accounts receivable, referral, and treatment tracking). In addition to compatibilities the software package must have a technical support system that is responsive and understands information technology (IT) infrastructure and the importance of the software to a functioning OMS practice. It is the author's experience that Oral Surgery Exec offers these features at a reasonable cost.

With emergent technologies there should be the ability to adopt the use of tablet personal computers (PCs) and PDAs for remote use of desired data. In addition, the software package should be fully integratable with the imaging modality used in the practice. With continued development of cone beam technology this flexibility is essential (see later discussion).

Before investing in a particular software and hardware package it is imperative to obtain sound professional IT assistance, enabling proper design and installation with the desired compatibility of the system with the other available technologies to be incorporated into the office. A well-designed and integrated software and imaging system located properly within the office space helps the office be more efficient and productive. If constructed poorly, however, it increases stress and frustration for the surgeon, staff, and least desirable of all, the patient.

Incorporation of cone beam technology

One aspect of OMS practice that has seen the greatest advancement in recent years is imaging. With the incorporation of cone beam technology becoming more prevalent and its capabilities realized in practice, our ability to diagnose and plan treatment has improved dramatically. Although computerized tomography scans are not new, the availability and real-time access to this type of information once was not available. Now, in-office cone beam scanners are a superior adjunct to any practice (Fig. 6). These cone beam computerized tomography (CBCT) machines are far more accurate than traditional panoramic radiographs used routinely in practice today [3–6]. Traditionally, if a more detailed study was necessary the patient would have to be scheduled for a CT scan at a local hospital or outpatient

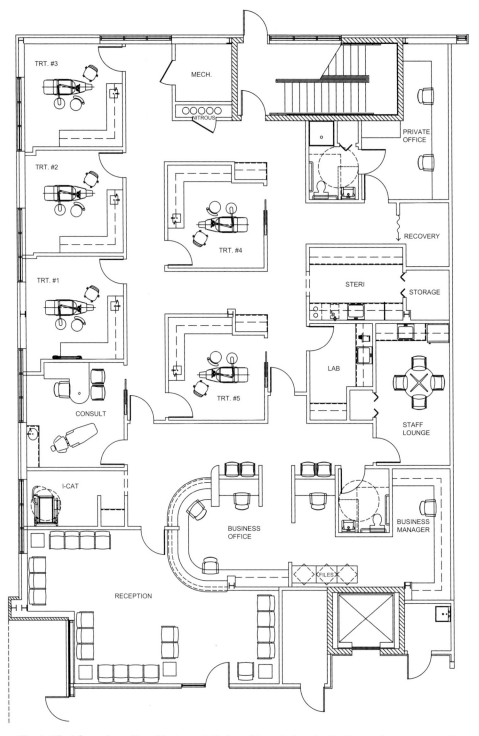

Fig. 5. Final floor plan with cabinetry and chair positions designed with discussed zones as a guide.

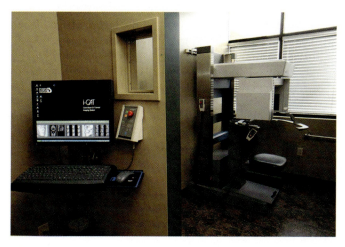

Fig. 6. Imaging room with CBCT scanner and designated work station with operator protection and visualization shown.

imaging center and then scheduled to follow up for the results and further consultation. Incorporating a cone beam scanner allows the surgeon to diagnose and plan treatment while the patient is present at the initial appointment and to truly understand and appreciate any relevant anatomic considerations necessary to complete treatment safely. Another important consideration is the reduced radiation dosing to the patient that a cone beam scanner offers compared with a traditional CT scanner [7–9]. Although an entire article could be dedicated to this new technology, discussing the intricate details of the machine and its capabilities, this discussion remains focused on its incorporation into the modern OMS practice.

In the near future, any new office design or floor plan will come standard with a room designated for a cone beam scanner. This equipment will only become more affordable as other manufacturers enter the market. Also, the machines will be designed with decreased radiation dosing, which is already more than acceptable. The file sizes will become more compressed allowing faster e-mail transmission and uploads into the electronic medical records of major software companies. The machines will also decrease in size and will offer faster image processing.

The current space requirement is generally not different than that for a standard panoramic/cephalometric machine but requires the use of a computer terminal to run and store images for further processing. This work station should allow visualization of the patient during the scan yet provide the appropriate shielding of the operator (see Fig. 6). This requires a shielding plan based on projected workload and proximity to personnel and patients. Based on use, lead shielding may be necessary around the imaging room. Incorporating this detail in the planning of the space or a remodeling project helps reduce expensive construction changes if there is an increase in use of the machine in the future.

This technology, when incorporated into the OMS practice, offers a true three-dimensional understanding of the anatomic relationships that exist, helping establish safe and reliable treatment plans efficiently. CBCT scans enable superior treatment counseling for third molar, implant, orthognathic, impacted teeth, and oral and maxillofacial pathology patients because there is no longer any guesswork as seen with two-dimensional imaging (Figs. 7 and 8) [3,6,8–12]. As this technology continues to advance the radiation dosing that currently is acceptable will continue to be reduced and the size of the machine will certainly be reduced. The integration of these images into the electronic medical record should also be condensed to allow easy, fast importation of images into the patient's chart. The incorporation of CBCT into OMS practice and implant dentistry will soon be standard of care and for the contemporary OMS this technology will enable more diagnoses and safer care (Fig. 9).

Necessary personnel

The generation of a modern OMS practice that is capable of paperless interaction with patients, insurance companies, and referrals is not an easy task. We have discussed some key elements that

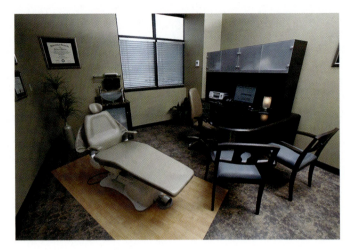

Fig. 7. Multiple views of a formal consultation room that is less clinical and allows a conference-style case presentation setting yet enables capability for a clinical exam.

help in relation to general layout, computer software needs, design, and technology, but probably the most important element is a team approach.

Initially one should enlist an IT person or team familiar with medical and dental office needs who can help coordinate and integrate particular software and hardware packages with the layout of the office and the associated technologies (ie, imaging equipment, tablet PCs, PDAs, and so forth). For example, you would not want to purchase imaging equipment that could not integrate with the patients' electronic medical records or have a system in place to allow the image to be present at the time of surgery or consultation. This team should also work in conjunction with the architect to allow proper positioning of monitors or work stations for staff to alleviate a shortage during patient check-in, treatment, or checkout. Coordinating the technological needs with the general structure during development it decreases problems once practice starts.

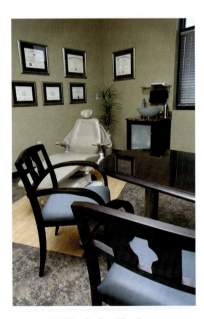

Fig. 8. See Fig. 7.

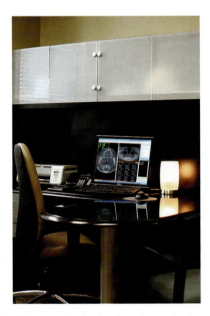

Fig. 9. Work station in the formal consultation room for CBCT manipulation and treatment planning at eye level with the patient.

The practice should work with architects who are familiar with the needs of this type of office design, encouraging the development of a functional space that offers appropriate, efficient flow for staff and patients. An experienced interior designer offers the ability to incorporate colors and accents to the space that help market the practice and do not detract from the expected level of care.

The unification of architect, designer, IT personnel, and practitioner either in the development of or transition to a technologically advanced office design helps realize the goal. Allowing these trained professionals to collaborate for a final product decreases the overall stress on the surgeon, avoiding the potential for regret and the need to make expensive changes in the future.

Practice marketing

Paying attention to details, such as floor plan, software packages, imaging modalities, and office interior, can be one of the most effective marketing tools for the practice. An office that is inviting based on color choice and decorating helps establish the practice as advanced in the initial impression of patients and referring doctors. Opening the new office (or a newly remodeled existing practice) and inviting patients or referring doctors to an open house is a great first step in creating a positive marketing campaign.

One technique to increase awareness of a practice is to develop a seminar schedule for local referring doctors sponsored by the practice, allowing the surgeon to share new and advance techniques and familiarizing the referral base with the particular skill set of the practice. The seminars can occur through a presentation-style format with lectures and guest lectures, or through journal/study clubs incorporating continuing education credit rewards for attendance.

The development of an identifying marker or logo for the practice used consistently on letterhead, business cards, and other marketing tools over time creates awareness among the public and referrals for the practice. This logo can be as simple as the practice's name or a detailed artistic symbol. No matter the logo, staying consistent with the mark over time helps create a synonymous link to the practice.

Marketing in the newspaper and local regional papers can often be expensive and determining the readership before planning an ad is important. Print advertising should be run in publications with the target audience in mind, not just the publication with the largest number of readers. If possible, continued placement in the same location with consistent messaging works better that random one-time advertising. The degree of artwork and size of the ad depends on the budget available.

The region in which one practices dictates which media channel offers the greatest return. For example, more rural practices may gain better exposure by marketing in a local newspaper, whereas in a major metropolitan area, an area or neighborhood monthly paper may be of greater benefit. A Web site designed to feature the practice and the services available is now routine. This type of access to on-line forms for pre-registration and questions helps streamline the office practice and allows the patient a first impression before entering the physical structure.

Overall marketing of the contemporary OMS practice should highlight those characteristics that set the practice apart. Highlighting capabilities such as CBCT technology and on-line registration helps create awareness of the type of availability and advanced care that is possible. The attention certainly should be directed toward patients, but given the referral nature of OMS through general dentists and other specialists the referring dental community should be a large target for any marketing campaign.

Summary

The modern OMS office holds unlimited potential for incorporation of many different technologies. The goal, however, should focus on establishing a facility and environment that is inviting to patients and ergonomically designed for safe and efficient care delivery for the surgeon and staff with an overall reduced level of stress. The possibilities in office design and incorporation of emergent technologies, imaging equipment, and media platforms continue to advance, allowing future OMS offices exciting possibilities in day-to-day operation.

References

[1] Wolkenhauer D. Joyce Bassett DDs smiles by choice. Catalyst 2007;1(1):12–20.
[2] Tholen M. Principles of floor planning. In: A guide to designing the elegant dental or medical office...the largest marketing tool of your career. 2005. p. 16–37.
[3] Tantanapornkul W, Okouchi K, Fujiwara Y, et al. A comparative study of cone-beam computed

tomography and conventional panoramic radiography in assessing the topographic relationship between the mandibular canal and impacted third molars. Oral Surg Oral Med Oral Pathol Oral Radiol Endod 2007;103(2):253–9.

[4] Hashimoto K, Arai Y, Iwai K, et al. Comparison of a new limited cone beam computed tomography machine for dental use with a multidetector row helical CT machine. Oral Surg Oral Med Oral Pathol Oral Radiol Endod 2003;95:371–7.

[5] Peck JL, Sameshima GT, Miller A, et al. Mesiodistal root angulation using panoramic and cone beam CT. Angle Orthod 2007;77(2):206–13.

[6] Closmann J, Schmidt BL. The use of cone beam tomography as an aid in evaluating and treatment planning for mandibular cancer. J Oral Maxillofac Surg 2007;65(4):766–71.

[7] Winter AA, Pollack AS, Frommer HH, et al. Cone beam volumetric tomography vs. medical CT scanners. N Y State Dent J 2005;71(4):28–33.

[8] Danforth RA, Dus I, Mah J. 3-D volume imaging for dentistry: a new dimension. J Calif Dent Assoc 2003;31(11):817–23.

[9] Nakagawa Y, Kobayashi K, Ishii H, et al. Preoperative application of limited cone beam computerized tomography as assessment tool before minor oral surgery. Int J Oral Maxillofac Surg 2002;31(3): 322–6.

[10] Lascala CA, Panella J, Marques MM. Analysis of the accuracy of linear measurements obtained by cone beam computed tomography (CBCT-NewTom). Dentomaxillofac Radiol 2004;33(5):291–4.

[11] Scarfe WC, Farman AG, Sukovic P. Clinical applications of cone beam computed tomography in dental practice. J Can Dent Assoc 2006;72(1):75–80.

[12] Liu DG, Zhang WL, Zhang ZY, et al. Three-dimensional evaluations of supernumery teeth using cone-beam computed tomography for 487 cases. Oral Surg Oral Med Oral Pathol Oral Radiol Endod 2007;103(3):403–11.

Marketing the Oral and Maxillofacial Surgery Practice Through Positive Employee Relations

Joe Niamtu III, DMD

Oral/Maxillofacial & Cosmetic Facial Surgery, 10230 Cherokee Rd. Richmond, VA 23235, USA

Marketing the oral and maxillofacial surgery practice

I have written numerous articles and textbook chapters on this subject, and it is impossible not to repeat aspects of my views on this subject. As medicine and society change, so does marketing. Some of this information is new, and some is verbatim from previous publications, but much of it is timeless and was probably realized by successful business people in ancient Rome. Marketing is a controversial word among doctors. Some practitioners embrace it and some disdain it, but one thing is for sure—we all market. Some of us market intentionally by exposing our indigenous patient population to information about our services while they sit in a bright, friendly waiting room, listen to a call-on-hold message, peruse brochures of our work, or are given exemplary service by well-trained staff. Others claim not to market yet expose their patients to negative marketing, such as dirty and crowded surroundings, long waits, rude receptionists, and poor practice management. Both of these scenarios involve marketing, even for doctors who say that they do not believe in marketing. The problem is that they are providing negative marketing. The underlying fact is that all doctors market, like it or not. The minute you unlock your door and roll your phones over in the morning, your marketing once again begins. Even when you are closed, you are marketing by the most powerful source of all, word of mouth.

The reputation of a practice never sleeps. Realizing this fact, the remainder of this article deals with the theories of superlative patient care through employee enhancement. I point out positive and negative influences in the world of marketing. I fully realize that this is one practitioner's opinion and others may differ, but these opinions have propelled our practice from a single oral and maxillofacial surgeon (OMS) with two employees to a nine-doctor group with seven offices and more than 50 employees. We are far from perfect and do not proclaim to hold the keys to the marketing universe, but we have come to realize and appreciate what works and have learned from our mistakes on what did not. Hundreds of OMSs around the country have found a balance of how to attract and keep patients and enjoy their profession. They also could easily write this article, and I have learned from many of them. The first rule of marketing is to always be a teacher and a student.

Employee relations

I have been an active and prolific practitioner of oral and maxillofacial surgery for 24 years. I have been lucky to have chosen eight partners who continued to drive our vision to the top and build their lives around the wonderful profession. I also have had the pleasure to befriend hundreds of other successful OMSs around the world. I truly believe if you ask average OMSs what are the best and the worst things about their practice, they will answer the question with one word: employees. The relationships you forge with your staff can produce some of the most rewarding experiences of your life. On the other hand, they can be the largest focus of stress in your life and potentially ruin your career. This range from great to horrible is not circumstance but is usually poor leadership on the part of the

E-mail address: niamtu@niamtu.com

doctor. As I write this article I am aware of employee problems within our practice that are mundane and common, although stressful and unproductive. At the same time, I am aware of several truly tragic situations involving friends of mine around the country. In one instance, a truly brilliant surgeon lost his license for writing prescriptions to his receptionist. Another friend has had his life and practice ruined from a sexual harassment suit. Still another friend suffered a huge lawsuit for actions of his employees. Because all of this information is fresh in my mind, I devote this article to employee relations. If you hire and train the right employees, marketing is almost automatic and the inverse is true. To establish a successful marketing practice, you must hire and train the right employees and terminate the employees who are not upholding the vision of your practice.

Because many new practitioners are reading this article, I begin at an elementary level and progress. The basis of the article is paramount to all employers regardless of the time in practice. Universal situations exist that enhance or detract from any business, and choosing the correct employees is paramount regardless of the type of business. This fact applies especially to all service-oriented businesses, of which health care happens to be. Unfortunately, many doctors never grasp the concept that their business is based on service and struggle and endure unnecessary stress while their colleagues who do understand the concept have fulfilling and profitable practices.

In any service-related industry, it is usually the level of service that sets businesses apart. For instance, if you had to ship one of your most prized possessions somewhere overnight and were ultimately concerned about its safe and timely arrival, would you choose Federal Express or the US Post Office? Most people would choose the former because of perceived level of customer service on behalf of Federal Express and the lackadaisical attitude often attributed to government agencies. Service of one's customer or patient base is the key to success. A doctor may be a genius and the best surgeon in a given area, but if the staff are abusing patients, the practice will not prosper (Box 1). On the other hand, a mediocre doctor can be elevated to hero status by a staff that nurtures their patients. Most doctors are clueless on correct hiring and firing concepts, and the ones with experience often have earned their knowledge through hard knocks. When I lecture to large groups of doctors in any locality,

Box 1. The 1995 American Society for Quality survey on the reasons customers switch service providers

- Death (1%)
- Moved away (3%)
- Influenced by friends (5%)
- Lured away by competition (9%)
- Dissatisfied with work (14%)
- Attitude of indifference on the part of an employee (68%)

employee relations always occupy one of the top three lists of practice stress.

In the past, poor hiring and termination practices may have meant only increased employee turnover and doctor stress. In the current litigious environment, improper human resource skills frequently lead to lawsuits. Wrongful discharge, sexual harassment, discrimination, and other employment-related litigation is on the rise. For a suit-prone employee, the ability to win a hugely unreasonable settlement holds much better odds than a lottery ticket. Sexual harassment suits have been settled for millions of dollars for innocently intended gestures or actions. This is a frank reality of modern employment law and circumstances. This is the wrong arena in which to learn by mistake. Suits for sexual harassment are not covered by malpractice or umbrella insurance and are the responsibility of the defendant. Guilty or not, subsequent publicity can be damaging to the morale and reputation and pocketbook of the doctor. Because most OMS offices involve a male doctor with a female staff, the author strongly advises all new practitioners to thoroughly gain information about local and local employment laws.

Initially, a new OMS will more than likely require a staff of at least three employees. The AAOMS recommends that two employees assist at surgery and someone tend to the front desk and clerical duties. Some new doctors may economize by using two employees and placing phones on a recorder during surgery; however, availability to referring doctors is compromised. There is no doubt that as soon a doctor can afford adequate staff, he or she will enjoy a safer and more efficient practice.

The easiest positions to fill are surgical assistants. A strong pool of dental assistants, nurses, and surgical techs exists. As with any business, previous experience is preferable. A seasoned assistant actually can teach many things to a new doctor. It is also preferable to hire an assistant who can obtain hospital assisting privileges. As with all positions, a friendly, compassionate, presentable, mature assistant is optimum. One potential problem of hiring new employees involves the age and experience levels of the applicant pool. This pay and experience level frequently abounds with young, inexperienced women, many of whom have little experience and whose reliability and maturity levels may be insufficient to suit one's needs. This segment of potential employees is often transient because of schooling, relationships, and childbearing. I have taken pride in hiring this type of employee and watching them grow into excellent staff members. This growth has been in the presence of superlative staff members who had the opportunity to mold the new employee into a polished employee. Hiring this type of person without the nurturing can lead to many employee/employer difficulties.

The job of practice receptionist is a much more challenging situation. This employee is literally the ambassador of the practice and, more than any other employee, can add or detract from the practice. This person is usually the first person who gives an impression of the spirit of your practice. In many cases, prospective patients call the office and are bounded by many barriers. Pain, expense, inconvenience, apprehension, third parties, and lack of appreciation of services are just some of the common barriers between a doctor and patients. Many of these patients are "shopping around" to find a caring and reassuring environment or the ability to tailor finances. An exceptional receptionist acts like a magnet to bring these patients into the practice, whereas a rude or noncompassionate person may distance them even more. This position calls for multitasking, especially for the new doctor with a small staff. Besides the receptionist duties, this employee must assist in coding, billing, insurance, accounts receivable, and collections. All of these functions are as vital to the success of the practice as the skill of the doctor. This position begs for a mature, experienced individual and commands a higher salary. This is money well spent, because this person literally can help shape the future of the practice.

Where to find good employees

This is a question posed by all businessmen and -women. Experience is important, and the optimum situation is to hire someone who has worked in an oral and maxillofacial surgery practice. I warn against hiring an employee from a colleague's office, unless it is discussed up front with the neighboring doctor. A new doctor can count on intimidating existing practitioners, and there is no need to start off in a deeper hole.

Local dental societies usually have newsletters with employment sections that can prove useful. The help wanted ads in the local paper are a traditional means of finding employees. I warn against placing anyone's home phone in the ad for applicants. It is not unusual to have many, many calls at all hours of the day and night. Instead, I suggest a neutral address or PO Box number for which to send resumés. If the new doctor does not have hiring experience, I suggest that a qualified party assist in the interview process. It is important to hire someone with the correct "fit" who will augment the personality of the doctor. Many employment situations are a roll of the dice, but I caution against hiring someone who conveys feelings of suspicion. This is no place for a demure introvert. Hire someone with good eye contact, a good smile, and an enthusiastic attitude. An employee who "glows" is a keeper and infects the other employees and patients with that glow.

As the practice prospers, additional employees will be added. It is not unusual for an OMS practice to have three to six employees per doctor. As I allude to later in this section, many offices feel that they are understaffed when they are actually overstaffed.

New doctors are frequently in a quandary as to starting salaries. By surveying colleagues in the general dental community, one can establish a scale for given positions in a given community. Many of the "throw away" dental periodicals offer yearly regional staff salaries and regional fees. One of the major incentives for many people to work is obtaining insurance benefits. In the health care professions, health insurance as a benefit is pretty much a given. Although there are many means of doing this, some of the most common are as follows. Many companies offer group health plans at a substantial savings, whereas other employers give their staff a monetary sum for the employee to use the plan of their choice. Because many employees may have coverage from spouses, they may not need all the benefits that another employee would. So-called "cafeteria plans" present a menu of options from which employees may choose and are a popular option. Other benefits include sick leave, holidays, uniform allowance, and retirement benefits. Most doctors have pension and profit-sharing plans and are required to match funds for employees. This is a tremendous benefit and is often overlooked. An employee with longevity can save thousands of dollars in 401 K plans or similar vehicles. This benefit must be fully explained to be appreciated and extends the gift of ownership to one's staff.

Let us direct our attention to the actual art and science of hiring and firing. If there is one element of running a business for which most doctors are unprepared, it is finding, keeping, and terminating employees. Almost every seasoned practitioner bears some emotional scar from improper handling of employee issues. Many in our ranks have been parties to lawsuits for violating the most basic tenets of employment procedures. Enumerating several commandments of hiring, it is important to discuss some absolute basics. Many of these principles probably existed in the marketplaces of ancient Rome, yet millions of bosses make these mistakes 2000 years later.

I feel strongly that it is an absolute infraction to hire spouses or family members as employees. Nepotism will, at some time, cause employee problems. I have lectured all over the country on this subject and am often met with resentment for stating this opinion. It never fails that at the end of a lecture a doctor or spouse confronts me in stern disagreement. My response is that there are always exceptions to the rule, but the doctor is aware of countless problems involving family. This is especially difficult for partners or other employees because preferential treatment may be perceived. The spouse also may have the "coach's son syndrome" and apply stresses that are unnecessary. There is no doubt that it is difficult for a partner or manager to reprimand one's spouse, and if push comes to shove, it is rarely the other person who must leave the practice. I have observed many state-of-the-art practices over the past 20 years, and it is rare to find an exceptional practice with family members as employees. Two exceptions that exist are having family help at the inception of the practice as a cost-saving issue or casual summer employment for odd jobs. While on the subject of nepotism, it is also an unwise practice to hire relatives of current staff. The same pitfalls apply, and many embezzlement schemes have involved this type of situation.

Although it seems painfully obvious, professional doctor-employee relationships should stay just that. In this era of sexual harassment, even the most benign of gestures can be grounds for a successful suit. I am aware of multiple cases throughout the country involving expensive and embarrassing outcomes for a surgeon. I am also aware of suits brought forth for telling off-color jokes, inappropriate body contact that involved "backrubs," and commenting on an employee's attire or physical traits. Another common violation is the temptation to manipulate monetary funds. Some doctors may pocket cash that comes across the front desk and feel that it is untraceable. Always remember that if a staff member witnesses a doctor evading taxes or doing anything illegal for that matter, he or she now has a partner. If the doctor can steal cash and no one knows, then why shouldn't the employee?

Doctors spend as much or more time with staff than they do with their family, and there exists a temptation to bare one's soul. I cannot stress enough the need to always keep some distance from the doctor's private life and what the employee knows or hears. The author is familiar with several exceptional surgeons who were dragged through the mud by terminated and disgruntled employees. Never underestimate the diabolic nature of scorned employees. Like in a nasty divorce, they use any weapon of destruction, so do not provide them with ammunition.

This section discusses hiring and the interview process. There is a true art to being a good interviewer. It involves the art of listening—listening to what an employee says and being able to read between the lines as to what the employee represents. I elaborate on this later. First, the dress and demeanor of an interviewee is important. Because most people are at their best dress and behavior at an interview, it is usually safe to assume that what you see is the best you will ever see. If dress or demeanor is inappropriate at an interview, it can only go downhill. I feel strongly about hiring bubbly, enthusiastic employees, and if applicants do not smile and show strong eye contact, they are usually a poor choice. An additional caveat involves an applicant who speaks negatively of previous employers. This behavior should be a severe warning, especially for individuals who claim to be "victims." There is little doubt that you will be the next bad guy on their list.

Experience should be high on the list of employment attributes. Training someone to do a job is OK, but for a new doctor it merely adds additional stresses. It is better to hire a "teacher" than a "student" for the new doctor. Interviews need not be exhaustive and should be standardized. In short, you have two people sizing each other up. Do not forget, applicants are also interviewing you as a boss, and when employees resign, they are effectively firing you as a boss. It is a two-way street. One good question to ask is what applicants liked or disliked about their previous job, which can extract key information about how an employee may interface in your office. It is important to know if they can meet your standards in terms of overtime and Saturdays.

The next most important thing is being able to relate your vision and the goals of your practice. You must present written documentation of who you are, where you are going, and how you plan to have an applicant assist your journey. Many doctors do not have these guiding principles in writing, and how can an employee relate to goals that are nonexistent? Again, you should provide applicants with their job description and discuss it in detail. If you desire an exceptional practice, you need to employ exceptional people. If you do not have written job descriptions, you must settle for mediocrity. I suggest that the doctor make an audio- or videotape that contains the guiding principles and visions of the practice, which standardizes the interview process and simplifies this task.

If you have properly defined your goals and visions, you can effectively ask employees if they want to play on your team and follow your rules. If you have not defined the rules of the game, then how can you possibly expect employees to play? I have presented the rules of the game to applicants, and they stated that they could not comply with our expectations. Such employees have done both of us a tremendous service because it may have been months of frustration before an employee quit or was terminated. The point is that if we did not have the job description and rules of the game defined, then we could not have gained this information.

Employee references can be patronizing or significant as to hiring. Unfortunately, legal precedents have been set and it can be grounds for a suit. Many employers are happy to get rid of a problematic employee and do not want to have any backlash from a bad reference, so their word may not be accurate. On the other hand, an employer may be afraid to give an accurate reference because of legal recourse. It probably requires speaking to several individuals to actually obtain an accurate base. To simplify this process, it is important to ask previous employers if they would hire an employee again. It is also prudent to ask them if the applicant possessed the attributes or lack thereof that we are about to discuss. This at least gives some standardization to the referral process and allows new employers to find out an applicant's ability to fit into their office. Any employer must be careful about providing a negative reference. If an applicant can prove that you have prevented them from employment, you may be liable. Million-dollar lawsuits have been awarded to employees who were able to prove defamation. The author severely cautions any employer against giving a verbal or written negative reference, especially to a stranger. Many large companies only verify employment history that an employee was hired on a given date and worked there for a given period of time. These companies refuse to comment on subjective questions. If an employer wants to provide a negative reference without jeopardizing himself or herself, the statement "I cannot comment on this employee under advice from my attorney" should make the point without creating liability.

There is no doubt that hiring the incorrect employee can cost thousands of dollars. The cost of training, loss of efficiency, and negative impact are immeasurable, but they cost money and they cause stress.

I feel that eight attributes make a perfect employee. For the sake of measurement, we refer to a perfect employee as a "10." What we desire is to be able to screen for employees who are a "7" or above. The following attributes greatly assist this evaluation process (Box 2).

Competency and presentation

Competency is the foremost attribute required in the consideration of an employee. In any service-oriented business, customers or patients

---

Box 2. Key interview points to consider when interviewing potential employees

1. Competency and presentation
2. Unconditional commitment
3. Giving or taking
4. Offensive or defensive behavior
5. Superstar or team player
6. Joyous demeanor
7. Self-management
8. Learner

seek and expect a certain level of care and service. When people go to a nice restaurant, they know in advance that it will be expensive. For that expense they expect a high level of service (ie, prompt seating, polite treatment, accurate ordering, fast service, and attention to detail). A waiter who cannot meet those expectations is incompetent. If you order a rare steak and salad with dressing on the side and get a well-done steak and a salad drenched in dressing, that is incompetence. This incompetence will, across the board, cause unhappy customers and eventually harm the reputation of the owner. What is frustrating is that the restaurant owner may really have paid attention to detail. He or she may have a beautiful facility with ample parking, purchase only the finest ingredients, and hire the best chef in the area. Despite all the attention to detail, a single incompetent employee may shatter the dream of having a fine restaurant by negating attention to detail. There is a difference between inexperience and incompetence. If our waiter had a badge that stated "waiter in training," we would expect a lesser level of service. This employee may become an excellent waiter but should not be turned loose on the public without supervision.

Presentation is also an important factor to consider in our business. The discipline of oral and maxillofacial surgery involves cosmetics, aesthetics, and health. One of your most powerful marketing principles is the appearance of the doctor and staff. Slovenly, out-of-shape staff with yellow teeth or fingers from smoking or excessive body piercings or tattoos do not embody the image we are trying to convey. An obese employee who is bubbly and neat may be an asset, but someone with cellulite bulging from dingy polyester white scrubs does not assist your marketing efforts.

Unconditional commitment

Unconditional commitment is defined as commitment with the lack of conditions. The closest example that I can find is a resident in a training program. As residents, we could not allow anything to take precedence over our work. None of us would have dreamed of telling our program chair that we could not meet a deadline because we ate lunch and did not have time. We were in an environment in which lunch was not a priority, and our work took precedence. When we are called to the emergency room in the middle of the night, we cannot say "It's late, call me in the morning." These are examples of unconditional commitment.

Owners of businesses have much more impetus to be unconditionally committed because they reap more of the benefits or failures than do the employees. For this reason, it is rare to find this level of commitment in an employee. One thing about any society is that people identify and bond with cohesive organizational units that convey a common goal. Fraternities, sororities, social clubs, sports clubs, bowling leagues, scouting troops, and church groups are examples of situations in which people unite and develop sometimes extreme loyalties. There is usually little monetary incentive in these groups, and the point is that we are social animals and extend great efforts for "the cause." This same socialism extends into office settings; when employees bond and identify, they put forth great efforts for the good of the practice. When you have a good leader, clear-cut goals, and the correct employees, the ensuing product is a beautiful machine. Doctors who have exceptional and profitable practices probably are good leaders and have exceptional employees with a well-defined common goal.

Unconditionally committed employees perform within reason to accomplish the task at hand. Applicant who will not work overtime or on Saturdays or follow your rules of the game are only conditionally committed and do not meet our criteria. Finally, employees may be unconditionally committed to you and not your vision. If employees are only committed to you and you come into work with a poor attitude, then they also take on your attitude. If employees are committed to your vision, however, then they can pull you aside and remind you of your commitment to excellence and point out that your attitude on that particular day is not what your goals define.

Givers versus takers

People are either givers or takers. Givers are loving, compassionate people who truly enjoy giving of themselves. These people understand the win/win concept and fully realize that the more they give, the more they receive in return. These people exude a generosity that is not measured in physical gifts but more importantly in the subjective sense. These people give gifts of advice, time, compassion, empathy, and service. By now, you should be getting a picture of what it is that we want in an employee.

On the other hand, takers operate in the win/lose environment because for them to win, someone else must lose or look bad. These people reminded the teachers that they did not collect the homework assignments in school. Their means were not to serve as a reminder but rather to look good at the expense of others. This is a malignant personality trait and is manifested in all sections of culture. An OMS who refers to other OMSs as competitors instead of colleagues is another example of a taker. Persons who speak negatively about anything to enhance their own identity are takers. Givers would complement other persons on their efforts and then focus on those of their own. Although it is impossible to screen for this attribute in an interview, this behavior must be identified and these people removed from your staff. One bad apple can spoil the whole barrel. If, as an employer, you come across the "what's in it for me?" attitude, you must take action. If employees must have someone lose for them to win, guess who loses? The losers are the boss, the other staff, and the patients.

Offensive and defensive employees

By this categorization we are referring to one's ability to accept change. Change is the basis for all molecular structure, and all of life—from the subcellular level up—involves motion, change, and energy. If you examine successful people and successful practices, you see that they thrive on change. Change should breed excitement, but for many people it breeds fear and insecurity. If doctors are truly interested in approaching excellence, then they must continually change all aspects of their practice to increase efficiency and service. I challenge and reward my staff for changing. We look at our forms, policies, and furnishings and brainstorm, as a group, on how to improve them. Accepted employee suggestions are validated by monetary rewards.

Some employees are intimated by change and take the "if it ain't broke, don't fix it" attitude, which is poison in a motivated practice. Employees who accept and encourage change are termed offensive, whereas employees who fear and resist change are termed defensive. I recently made significant changes to the current charting system in my office. These changes meant altering the status quo of everyone's interaction in the structure and handling of the office charts. It was truly enlightening, as an employer, to witness the offensive staff immediately recognizing the potential for increased efficiency and service, whereas the defensive staff members could only see problems. For these defensive staff, it meant doing things differently, and although it was actually less work on their part, they resisted because of their personality traits.

It is appropriate for staff to challenge change. When I proposed the charting system changes, I did not consider some shortcomings and was enlightened by challenge from the offensive staff. It was interesting that the pitfalls put forth by the defensive staff were less founded to improving anything. We all like change because it counters boredom. If we all wore the same clothes every day and ate the same food at every meal, life would not be as interesting. The same holds true in the workplace. Valid leaders understand that all change may not be effective and must concede to their staff that a given plan was not working. It is acceptable to make mistakes and not dwell on them but rather move forward and, by trial and error, enhance the service to patients. Successful practices have offensive players.

Superstars versus team players

The term "superstar" is not a positive adjective in the sense we are using it. A superstar is the type of employee who can do it all. Although this might be appropriate or even desirable for your first employee, you will have problems when you begin adding staff. Superstars manipulate situations so all the attention swirls around them. It is not about winning the game; it is about how many points they scored. Superstars feel that for their previous experience or superior intellect they can "do better." They feel superiority and are often overprotective of the doctor and the practice. Their attitude is that they must "save" the practice from the incompetent hands of other employees. These employees may take some time to recognize, because they seem so dedicated on the surface. If one examines the attitudes of their co-workers, it becomes evident whether they are respected leaders and role models or self-servingly critical.

There are tricks to ferret out this personality type. Superstars frequently place themselves in situations that "no one else can do." For instance, they are the only ones who can back up the computer or the only ones who do the payroll. They thrive on being needed for important functions. They frequently do this to become indispensable. They may cause employee problems and realize that the other employee will be fired because the practice cannot run without the efforts of the superstar. You cannot fire these employees because no one else can perform the vital functions, such as back up or payroll. The key to neutralizing superstar status is cross-training. Give several staff responsibility for critical functions. This is good business sense and lessens the chance of fraud and embezzlement. Cross-training prevents superstardom.

These examples do not mean that one person should not have responsibility. The difference is in the person. Whereas superstars want other staff kept in the dark, team players communicate the important responsibilities to the other staff so that the office functions in their absence. Look for, hire, and reward team players, because they make your life and practice less stressful.

Although oral and maxillofacial surgery is not physically challenging, many doctors go home at night exhausted and stressed. They are not exhausted from doing surgery; they are exhausted from having to constantly manipulate staff members to keep peace. Superstars embezzle from the practice. They do not steal money, they steal energy. They are like sponges and they steal the energy and excitement from the other staff or even patients. To counter this type of behavior in these "indispensable" staff, the doctor must constantly manipulate situations and environment, which becomes stressful and exhausting. Surround yourself with team players and you will be energized. Synergy occurs when the total is greater than the sum of the parts. Team players, offensive staff, and givers blend harmoniously to cause synergy.

Enthusiasm, joy, and energy

Knowing that we spend a significant part of our time with our staff, it makes sense to seek enthusiastic, joyous, and energetic people. Happiness and enthusiasm are contagious and self-perpetuating. Friendly people with high energy levels are a welcome addition to any group of people anywhere. If you truly believe that there are no dress rehearsals in life, then you should make the most of every waking second. For movers and shakers there is no room for pessimism. The form of oral and maxillofacial surgery is not particularly exciting for the patient, but enthusiastic, joyous, energetic staff members can greatly enhance the service and happiness level of patients through attitude. Surround yourself with enthusiastic, joyous, energetic employees with the other previously mentioned attributes and your practice will prosper.

Self-management

Once you have found staff with positive attributes, you need to make sure that they are self-managing. Some employees know just what to do but do not perform unless directly supervised. This is a drain because you need two people to do the job of one. There is nothing wrong with the concept of a manager, but if you must literally stand over someone to ensure progress, you have an employee who is not self-managing. Self-managing employees are a pleasure to work with and take all the effort out of management.

Termination

If I could highlight a single entity that holds back progress and perpetuates turmoil, it would be the ignorance and hesitancy of doctors to terminate an employee. One must make a decision to run a practice or an employee repair service. There is no doubt that terminating an employee is a decision that is wrought with emotional and legal ramifications. Firing someone or being fired can provoke so many emotions in both parties that many doctors procrastinate or endure years of unnecessary stress because they cannot bring themselves to "pull the trigger."

In this situation, we ignore the tenets of big business. In the corporate world, termination and the factors leading to it are clearly defined, and it is not uncommon for employees to be terminated in the presence of co-workers while a company security guard hands them a box in which to place belongings and then escorts them to the door. It is traumatic for employees to be terminated because it signifies failure and humiliation. It is even worse when employees feel that they were unfairly terminated. If an employee is terminated for being tardy and has the retort that "Mary Ann is always late," your credibility is lost and you may open yourself for a wrongful termination suit. The best way to avoid termination is to use correct hiring principles. This sounds so trite, but in most offices hiring is such a haphazard event that it becomes a roll of the dice. In my travels I am constantly amazed by the lack of attention to basic human resource policy. Well-established offices often do not have written job descriptions, policy manuals, employee documentation files, and other basic information. Every office should have written policy on exactly what it takes to be an excellent employee and what it takes to be terminated. Employers also must be consistent with these policies with every employee. If employees do not know the goals of the practice, the day-to-day policies, and what is expected of them, how can they be expected to perform? Without structure one has chaos. Unfortunately, many practices—new and old—function in a chaotic state.

For these reasons, every practice needs a map and a compass. The map is the policy manual, and the compass is the leader of the practice, the doctor. No one can get from point A to point B in unfamiliar territory or inclement weather without navigational aids. Can you imagine a football team with no one designated as the quarterback? If there was no leader and anyone could call any play at any time, chaos would rule and the team would never advance. Similarly, if the team had a quarterback who knew all the plays but had no playbook for the rest of the team, the same chaos would rule. Any successful team must have a leader and a playbook, and any pilot must have a map and a compass. Similarly, every office must have a leader and rules of the game, which are mentioned later.

When the performance of an employee begins to falter, the leader must conscientiously ask himself or herself if it is an employee or employer problem. The perceived employee problem is often actually a leadership problem. If it is truly an employee problem and the employee can be salvaged, then a written warning and a second chance may be extended for a probationary period. If the employer feels that the employee is not catching on or is unsalvageable, then it is better to approach the inevitable as soon as possible. It is also important to document employee shortcomings and proof of counseling the employee, which is critical in terms of defending a wrongful discharge suit or an unemployment claim.

The task of termination

If the proper pre-termination steps have been performed, the actual task of termination need not be complicated. The single most important point is to have the entire script well thought out and clear in your mind. This is no time to ad lib or fumble around; absolute clarity is essential. It is also important to realize that if you are unhappy with the performance of a staff member, he or she is probably aware of it and is probably unhappy. Sometimes the termination of employment is actually a relief to both parties. I always terminate an employment relationship on a Friday afternoon, unless a significant infraction, such as theft or substance abuse, has transpired. It is important to have a private environment away from other employees, and it is mandatory to have an employee, preferably of the opposite sex, present to document and witness. I simply tell an employee that the employment relationship is not working. I further tell the employee that I think he or she is a fine person but not a good fit for the practice. I state that I have a certain vision and direction for the practice and that the employee is not moving toward the goals of the practice, which is not a good fit. I prefer not to delve into specifics because it opens the door for argumentation or comparison to other employees. If the employee pushes in that direction, I take control of the situation and reiterate that the topic is not open for discussion and move on. It is imperative not to insult an employee and leave him or her with poor self-esteem. If the situation is applicable, I offer the employee the ability to resign with severance benefits or be terminated with no benefits. I enter the interview with two predrafted letters—one for resignation and one for termination—and give the employee a choice. If I feel that there may be legal implications or retribution, I have the practice attorney present. It is acceptable to have a manager or attorney do the actual firing, as long as the proper channels are followed. It may be wise for the doctor to distance himself or herself from these proceedings and stick to doctoring. I have eight partners and more than 50 employees. Because of the size of our practice, we have an administrator with medical group management experience and a trained and experienced human resources manager. Hiring and firing are ongoing occurrences and are beyond the scope and training of the doctors.

Although it may seem cold, it is an absolute necessity to obtain any keys, credit cards, or any other practice possessions immediately. There are many cases of documented sabotage involving the lack of following this protocol. An even greater temptation for sabotage is to terminate an employee with 2 weeks' notice, which is a perfect invitation for the person to be unproductive or diabolic within your office. A prudent employer already has a replacement lined up for the position. I stated earlier that some doctors commit serious errors in judgment by taking money from the front desk, having affairs with staff, or allowing staff to know personal or family information. After being fired, an employee may become disgruntled and expose any deceit or retribution, which is a real and all too common situation. Do not fall victim.

Putting it all together through communication

I have outlined many theories and techniques related to marketing and patient service. I have used the phrase "content, happy and profitable practice" many times throughout this article. Anyone who has built this type of office can testify that it is a task of significant proportion, and the pursuit of excellence is never ending. It is said that excellence is a journey, not a destination, because there is no finish line. If someone is truly dedicated to the profession and practicing with enjoyment and profitability, then he or she will pay attention to the following tenets:

- Hire and maintain the correct staff
- Provide leadership and enthusiasm
- Make clear what is expected through a policy manual
- Train the staff to be patient-centered service providers
- Reward them for their efforts
- Pursue excellence in all facets of your practice
- Know when to terminate an employee
- Constantly improve the level of training and communication
- Always be a teacher and a student

These tenets are key to setting the stage for organized marketing. Without them, there is no marketing, unless it is negative marketing. A common misconception is that marketing merely involves the physical techniques mentioned earlier. A surgeon cannot market alone, and an uninformed or undertrained staff cannot market at all. Constant communication and consultation are paramount to keeping the team sharp. No football team would ever reach the championship without practice. For the OMS this practice involves staff communication. Any progressive practice has regular meetings with the doctors, managers, and staff. Although one's staff may know what to do and what to say, it must be continually stressed to stay aware and sharp. Enthusiasm is contagious, and the same may be said of the lack thereof. This team spirit must be perpetuated. I have monthly staff meetings with the partners and manager, quarterly staff meetings with everyone included, and an annual retreat for staff focused on communication, patient service, and continuing education. The manager also has regular meetings with various locations. One does not need to have a group to do this. In fact, it is much easier with a smaller office. Regardless of size, everything in this article applies to all offices.

To enhance communication, one must have policy and consistency in all positions. My partners and I have used a set of communication principles we refer to as "The Rules of the Game." This is an excellent list from which to build and a valuable tool to show a prospective employee that you are contemplating hiring. Every game has rules, and to win, one must be acutely aware of all the rules to avoid a disqualification. The winners in oral and maxillofacial surgery are happy, profitable practices, and the losers are those who go home exhausted and frustrated and dislike what they do for a living.

The following principles are referred to as the "Rules of the Game," and in my office they take precedence over all other forms of communication. All partners, managers, and employees are aware of the rules and they are posted throughout the office in bright, laminated frames. I feel that it is important for each person in the practice to have an intimate knowledge of the rules, and like referees in sports, the owners and managers must have an even greater understanding. The following sections examine each rule and its implication as it relates to oral and maxillofacial surgery.

Be willing to support our missions, values, and guiding principles

This rule, although obvious, is the most often overlooked. I am amazed and confounded by how many OMS practices do not have a written policy manual with distinct job descriptions and a clear outline of the vision or goals of the practice. If you do not communicate these with employees, how can you possibly expect them to support them?

Speak with good purpose

Gossip among doctors and employees is one of the most destructive forces in an office. It involves speaking about someone outside of his or her presence. Gossip is spoken by idle, unchallenged employees and can undermine your entire staff and effort. It should be grounds for termination and strictly prohibited. This also applies to those who say one thing and do another. Leaders must truly practice what they preach. Like your mom said, "If you can't say anything nice, don't say anything!" This especially holds true for pessimists.

Be open and honest in your communication with each other

Actually expressing one's true feelings is sometimes difficult. We are often afraid to hurt someone's feelings, rock the boat, or cause friction, so often it is easier to agree with someone or support improper behavior because you may be intimidated to express the truth. This is one of the most difficult things for some people to do, but if this rule is not followed, the others are meaningless. One must be able to look partners, managers, and employees in the eye and tell them exactly how they feel. If this is done with consistency, a person will be respected. For this to work, all individuals must take a pledge to be open and honest. It breaks the ice and paves the way for open-ended communication. Failure to do so perpetuates the problems of communication that plague many practices.

Complete agreements and be responsible to others and yourself

When people try to iron out problems, it is human nature for everyone to want to jump on the bandwagon and volunteer to take responsibility for making a change, which frequently involves a task, behavior change, or sacrifice. All too often, people who are enthusiastic starters often lose their vigor or neglect to follow through on the task or the promised behavior. This fault is common and is one huge reason why some practices never get out of the hole. It is imperative that when people say they will do something, they take the responsibility to follow through and the leader of the practice takes the responsibility to coach them through the stated work and insist on its timely completion. People must realize that when they fail to follow through on a task, they let themselves and the practice down.

1. Make only agreements that you are willing and intend to keep.
2. Clear up any broken or potentially broken agreements at the first appropriate time with the appropriate person, which is especially important. If one sees that a person is missing the promise or timeline, it is important to discuss this with the correct person at the correct time. The immediate leader for this staff position must be made aware of the possible lack of follow through and it should be expressed immediately. Complaining to the incorrect person may be gossip, and failing to notify the leader immediately compounds the problem by procrastination.
3. Do not commit to others unless there is agreement. Simply because a given individual feels that he or she has the correct idea or action does not make it correct. This fact must be clearly communicated to the group and a positive response must ensue, which requires rule number 3.

If a problem arises, look first at the system, not the people, and then make the correction

If there is one thing that many employers are guilty of it is this. I stated earlier that most employee problems are the result of the employer, not the employee, which is usually true. Employees often take the brunt of criticism when the employer is guilty of being a poor leader. If there are no policy manuals, job descriptions, vision, or goals, then whatever occurs is happenstance or coincidence. Your chances of having an enjoyable, profitable practice fall into the odds of winning the lottery. Virtually any employee problem can be traced to improper leadership. Next time you are disappointed with an employee, stop and look in the mirror and ask yourself as a leader, "Did I do everything possible to make the rules and goals known and set clear standards to be followed in this case?" It takes a big person, but so often a leader cannot answer this question in the affirmative. A true leader admits shortcomings and does better; a poor leader continues to be a blamer.

Do not be a blamer

No one likes taking criticism or being wrong, but blaming others for one's failure or shortcomings only perpetuates mediocrity. The three hardest words to say are "I was wrong." Once a person can speak with honesty and admit the failure, he or she will be respected and open the door for other individuals to exhibit this honesty. For this environment to exist, the other staff must be supportive and accept apology and honesty and not persecute the individual or dwell on the admission.

Commit to add value by making more out of less

For any business to thrive, each person must add value. Stress and waste occur when staff or doctors detract value. The key to operating a successful business in this day of managed care and business is to be lean, economical, innovative, and value conscious, not only in physical spending but also on decisions and the entire aura of the practice. Waste in policy or expenditures severely affects the ability for some doctors to enjoy their work and make a profit. Each staff member should constantly challenge the others and the practice to do more with less, and when a suggestion is valid, that employee should be rewarded.

Have the willingness to win and allow others to win

In a win/win situation, the attitude is "if I allow others to win, then I win also." With an employer, the win is even bigger. This is a competitive world, and many people are used to winning to be promoted or to advance. Unfortunately, many of these people feel that they can win only if someone else loses, which creates a backstabbing environment; for the person to win, someone must lose. If this person is your employee, then the practice ultimately loses. These people are goal oriented and difficult to control. On the other hand, win/win employees progress and advance just as fast and with fewer waves because they realize that by allowing others to win, they win and may win bigger. This type of employee portrays altruism and is a valuable asset to any practice. The world needs more winners.

Focus on what works and retreat on what does not

Often the best intentions are put forth with ideas or policies, only to have them fail or fall short of the intended benefit. A progressive leader realizes that some ideas, no matter how good they seem, are not feasible. These leaders admit the shortcoming, regroup, and attack the problem from another angle. A poor or resistant leader does not admit to the shortcoming and beats a dead horse, although it is not in the best interest of the practice. Some leaders remain hardheaded and propagate poor policy because they cannot admit to being incorrect. No matter how good it sounds, if it does not work, move on. What is also important is not to focus too much on the past. If one is surrounded by individuals who do not forget a mistake and continually reflect on what did not work, the proper environment is not being fostered to admit a mistake. Do not dwell on the past; learn from mistakes and move on.

Encourage the risk of innovation

One must focus on the best communication for staff and the best service and care for patients. Doing this requires going outside of the usual parameters for practice and service. If one follows the usual details for running a practice, then one will have a usual practice. To have an exceptional practice, one must constantly challenge the leaders and the staff to think of innovative means to better the communication and patient service and care. Sometimes staff are shy or hesitant to provide input. Sometimes people who provide input are ridiculed or ignored or, worse yet, go unrewarded. Big business learned decades ago that it pays to have good ideas and one should pay for good ideas. If employees make a suggestion that makes a difference, they deserve reward. They win, you win bigger, and your patients win biggest.

An example is how our practice decreased after-hour calls by 90%. No one loves being on call and we all get nuisance calls. Many or most of the after-hour calls involve medications. Some calls are warranted and many are from drug seeking patients. Our practice simply put a message on our after-hours recorder that stated, "No prescriptions are filled after hours or on weekends." We also posted these signs throughout the office. We initially feared that we may offend legitimate patients in pain, but we were wrong. Legitimate patients called during office hours and drug seekers called someone else. We literally decreased our emergency calls by 90%.

Do not shoot the messenger

Upon hearing bad news, the king killed the messenger, as the story goes. None of us want to hear bad things about our practice, but to ignore them only makes things worse. Ignorance is bliss only for someone who wants to work in a stressful and nonprofitable environment. A good leader must demand to know what is good and what is bad and must liberate the staff, patients, and referring doctors to have unencumbered input. If you make it hard for someone to tell you negative things, you never hear them. This is not reality. Sometimes it requires a negative to make a positive. True leaders have an open-door policy for constructive criticism and act accordingly. Before criticizing someone, first try to understand the principles of the policy and always offer criticism in a positive and constructive manner, as stated in rule number 3. Encourage critique!

Raise the "red flag" when overloaded

Leadership requires energy, and sometimes—with the best of intentions—we put too much responsibility and burden on ourselves. Although we think we can handle it, we become overloaded and begin to break rule number 4. This behavior, although done with good intentions, actually encumbers the practice and skews all the rules. We all have limits of responsibility that we can handle and must maintain a good mix of relaxation and outside activities. If one becomes overloaded, in trying to make something better, he or she may actually make it worse. We all tend to multitask; sometimes instead of advancing a few prime goals we wallow in stagnation, which leads to inefficiency and burnout. If our managers "raise the flag," we can appreciate their honesty instead of admonishing them months later when we see that the projects are not done. It is more advantageous to admit overload and ask for help to keep the practice on track. Never be afraid ask for assistance and never create an environment in which this communication is frowned upon.

Always maintain a sense of humor

Life is a short ride, and we all have only so many heartbeats to enjoy it. Sometimes we take things way too seriously. There is a time for seriousness and a time for levity. Most influential and successful people with whom I have had the pleasure of being associated always find humor in life and make the best out of all situations. As OMSs, we live in a high stress environment and face sometimes grave decisions on a daily basis. No matter how bad things seem in a given crisis, history tells us that they will pass and improve. Optimism is a virtue and is contagious. Try to smile every second and find humor and laughter in life. There are no dress rehearsals in life! How would you treat people today if you knew it was your last day on earth? The button that fell off your shirt or the flat tire would carry much less aggravation.

Summary

This article was intended to be about marketing. Many readers may have appreciated more specific discussion on exact techniques or "how do I do it?" Those topics can be covered in a future article, but having superlative acumen on employee relations is much more important to all OMSs than "how to take a referring doc to lunch." Keep a copy of this article handy and distribute it to all new employees. Review the hiring and firing tenets and "Rules of the Game" each time you hire a new employee, fire an established one, or face trying times with staff or partners.

Acknowledgments

I would like to thank Howard Rochesti of the Mercer Corporation in Santa Barbara, California for his ability to distill the valuable information in Box 2 into simple categories.

Information and Computer Technology in Oral and Maxillofacial Surgery

Reena M. Talwar, DDS, PhD, Daisy Chemaly, DMD, FRCD(C)

Division of Oral and Maxillofacial Surgery, University of Toronto, 124 Edward Street, Room 148, Toronto, Ontario, Canada, M5G 1G6

Computer technology has become an integral part of the world we live in. It has not only advanced the areas of day-to-day communication and education but has taken the clinical world into a new realm of achievement. The Internet has been a beneficial and obstructive part of this growth process. The information available to the world, although abundant in nature, is sometimes poorly monitored or censored. Today's clinicians are required to be more and more adapted to the ever-changing technologies around us. Various diagnostic and planning tools have been available to us as clinicians in the treatment for our patients; however, it is the advancements in these areas through computer technologies that have provided an incredible advantage to the clinical world.

Diagnostic imaging has always been an integral part of the specialty of oral and maxillofacial surgery. The American Academy of Oral and Maxillofacial Radiology (AAOMR) has established "parameters of care" providing rationales for image selection for diagnosis, treatment planning, and follow-up of patients with conditions affecting the oral maxillofacial region, including temporomandibular joint (TMJ) dysfunction (parameter 2), diseases of the jaws (parameter 3), and dental implant planning (parameter 4) [1]. For most dental practitioners, the use of advanced imaging has been limited because of cost, availability, and radiation dose considerations [2]. Various imaging modalities have been used in the dentomaxillofacial fields over the past few decades, related to implant planning; TMJ imaging; detection of facial fractures, lesions, and diseases of soft tissues in the head and neck; and reconstructive craniofacial surgery [3]. Some of the more commonly used imaging modalities, such as plain films (periapical, occlusal, or panoramic radiographs) and conventional tomography, are limited in their diagnostic potential. These modalities provide the clinician with two-dimensional images that are often distorted and difficult to assess accurately. In situations in which a more precise and detailed image is necessary, the clinician has been limited to obtaining CT scans, oftentimes needing to outsource for this request. Depending on the type of practice and affiliation with a hospital, obtaining CT scan images can be an expensive and time-consuming process. Specific areas of advancement in the field of radiology have made such necessities less of a task for the clinician and the patient. In particular, the advent of cone beam CT has provided clinicians with a practical source for diagnosis and treatment planning for our patients. As with all imaging modalities, cone beam CT also has certain limitations, yet it provides the clinician with a three-dimensional model from which a larger amount of diagnostic data can be extracted and used.

Other areas of advancement in computer technologies related to oral and maxillofacial surgery are specific to the treatment planning phase of patient care. Numerous software programs have become available in the market in the areas of implantology, orthognathic surgery, and craniofacial surgery during the past decade. These software programs are allowing the clinician to plan the outcome of the surgical procedure on a virtual basis and, in some instances, to prepare the final prosthetic outcome for the patient before the actual surgical procedure. An example of this

E-mail address: r.talwar@utoronto.ca (R.M. Talwar).

type of software is the NobelGuide software planning program designed by NobelBiocare (Göteborg, Sweden). This software program, although similar in concept to the Simplant (Glen Burnie, Maryland) program, not only provides the clinician with a highly sophisticated virtual treatment planning computer program but allows for fabrication of the final/temporary prosthesis before surgery. From a conceptual point of view, this is, in fact, what the future of computer technology is all about. A focus on the diagnostic and treatment planning phase of patient care then allows for a decreased risk in the overall surgical procedure being provided, greater patient benefit, and a successful outcome in the long term.

The focus of this article is to provide the oral and maxillofacial surgeon with an overview of some of the recent information and computer technologies available in the marketplace as they relate to diagnostic imaging, implantology, orthognathic surgery, and craniofacial surgery. In so doing, the author hopes to highlight the various advantages and disadvantages of each of these technologies, and thus provide the clinician with a wider range armamentarium with which to treat his or her patient successfully and predictably.

Computer technology in diagnostic imaging

In 1994, i-CAT (Xoran Technologies, Ann Arbor, Michigan; Imaging Sciences International, Hatfield, Pennsylvania) launched cone beam CT as an alternative modality from conventional CT scanning for the dentomaxillofacial region. The need for such a system stemmed from the "gray zone" that existed in radiology between two-dimensional plain films and sophisticated conventional CT scans.

Cone beam CT provides highly accurate images with lower radiation exposure to the patient in a shorter amount of time. The added benefit of these systems is their overall reduction in cost, size of the unit, and positioning of the patient. In a conventional CT scan, the patient is traditionally in a supine position. Cone beam CT allows the patient to sit upright as he or she would for a standard panoramic radiograph (Fig. 1). This helps to alleviate some of the claustrophobia for patients, which is intrinsic to the conventional CT scanning protocol. Also, the fact that these units are much smaller in overall size and versatile with regard to their applications makes cone beam CT an up and coming standard modality for oral and maxillofacial surgical practice.

Cone beam CT scanners are based on volumetric tomography, using a two-dimensional extended digital array providing an area detector, which is then combined with a three-dimensional x-ray beam [2]. The patient is positioned upright, as in the case of obtaining a standard panoramic radiograph, with the head stabilized in a head holder or positioner. The scanner then performs a single 360° scan of the patient's maxillofacial region and collects single-projection images, known as "basis images," at various time intervals (Fig. 2). The concept of cone beam CT is similar to conventional CT in that images are manipulated by sophisticated algorithms that are incorporated into the imaging software program to generate a three-dimensional image of the patient that can be viewed in axial, sagittal, and coronal planes [2]. Some of the more commonly available systems include the NewTom QR DVT 900 (Quantitative Radiology s.r.l., Verona, Italy), CB MercuRay (Hitachi Medical Corporation, Kashiwa-shi, Chiba-ken, Japan), 3D Accuitomo-XYZ Slice View Tomograph (J. Morita Mfg Corporation, Kyoto, Japan), and i-CAT [2].

The documented advantages of this new technology for maxillofacial imaging include a reduction in the size of the irradiated area, improved accuracy of the image, rapid scan time, reduction in the dose of radiation delivered to the patient, less metal artifact, and ease of conversion of data for use with maxillofacial-related software [2]. Several investigators have revealed excellent image acquisition for different structures within the head and neck region, such as morphology of the mandible and location of the inferior alveolar nerve canal [4–6]. Kobayashi and colleagues [7] confirmed the superiority of the PSR 9000 cone beam CT (Asahi Roentgen, Kyoto, Japan) to spiral CT in terms of spatial resolution on cross-sectional images. The one clear advantage of cone beam CT over conventional CT scanners is its lower radiation dose to the patient; however, differences also exist between the various cone beam CT scanners available in the marketplace. In an article by Ludlow and colleagues [8], a direct comparison was made between two cone beam scanners, the i-CAT and the NewTom 3G (Quantitative Radiology) with respect to dosimetry values, and it was found that the dosimetry value of the i-CAT cone beam unit was 1.6 to 1.8 times higher than that of the NewTom 3G unit.

In a study by Hirsch and colleagues [9], five human cadaver heads were examined by spiral CT (Somatom Emotion; Siemens, Erlangen,

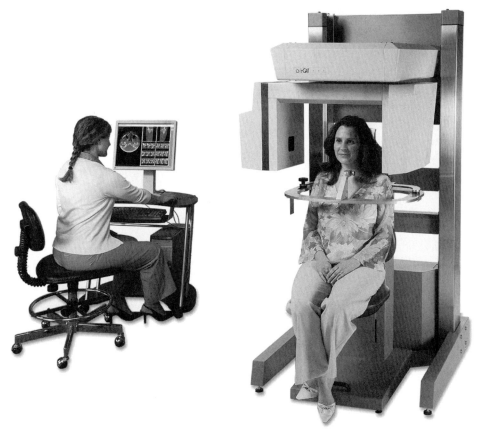

Fig. 1. i-CAT cone beam CT unit demonstrates upright positioning of the patient and an amorphous silicon flat-panel image sensor resulting in a sophisticated compact design. (*Courtesy of* Imaging Sciences International, Hatfield, PA; with permission.)

Germany), cone beam CT (NewTom DVT 9000) and the 3D Accuitomo. The quality of the image was evaluated by five different observers using a five-point rating scale. The results of this study indicated that the 3D Accuitomo cone beam scanner had the best image quality as compared with the NewTom D 9000 cone beam scanner and the spiral CT scanner.

Although there are obvious benefits to using cone beam CT over conventional CT scans, what are the advantages of this diagnostic modality over standard plain film radiographs? It is the responsibility of the clinician to know and be able to communicate the dose and selection of specific examinations to his or her patients. Earlier reports on cone beam CT radiation exposure to the patient indicated that the dose was equivalent to a few panoramic radiographs; however, this information was based a single vendor and a 9-inch field of view (FOV) [10]. More recently, other researchers have found that although full FOV doses from the dentomaxillofacial cone beam CT units are between 2% and 23% of the dose of comparable conventional CT examinations, they are also several to hundreds times greater than single panoramic image exposures [8,11]. Although in comparison to conventional plain radiographs, the cone beam examination provides the clinician with substantial additional information, it is the responsibility of the clinician to select the most appropriate radiographic examination based on the amount of detail information required for that particular patient.

The need for accuracy in implant placement became a driving force for the combination of diagnostic technology, such as cone beam CT and surgical implant planning software. Sarment and colleagues [12] compared the accuracy of a conventional implant surgical guide with that of a stereolithographic surgical guide using epoxy

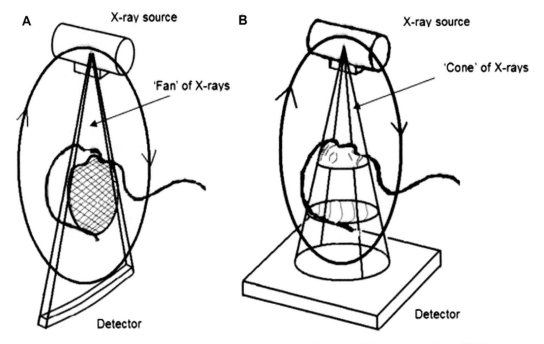

Fig. 2. X-ray beam projection scheme compares single-detector array fan beam CT (*A*) and cone beam CT (*B*) geometry. (*Adapted from* Scarfe WC, Farman AG, Sukovic P. Clinical applications of cone-beam computer tomography in dental practice. J Can Dent Assoc 2006;72(1):77; with permission.)

edentulous mandibles into which five implants were placed on each side of the jaw. The average distance between the planned implant and the actual osteotomy was compared after implant placement by comparing preoperative planning with postoperative placement. The average distance between the planned implant and the actual osteotomy was 1.5 mm coronally and 2.1 mm apically using the conventional surgical guide as compared with 0.9 mm and 1.0 mm, respectively, using the stereolithographic guide. Taking into consideration some of the obvious limitations of the study, it is still evident that the cone beam CT–based stereolithographic surgical guide provided the clinicians with a more precise planning modality for implant placement.

Computer technologies in implantology

Implantology has become a mainstay not only in the specialty of oral and maxillofacial surgery but in the field of dentistry as a whole. Implantology, as related to the implant fixtures, has been a rapidly advancing field of research and development. Changes in biomaterials and surface processing have allowed the clinician to change the protocol for implant surgery from a conventional staged procedure over a period of months to one that is more efficient and predictably successful. Not only have implants changed over the years, but the technology used to place implants from a diagnostic standpoint has advanced. As discussed previously in this article, the use of cone beam CT technology has provided the clinician with a three-dimensional model with which to plan implant placement more accurately. When combining this sophisticated diagnostic modality with virtual treatment planning software, the overall advantages are numerous.

The Simplant software system was the first three-dimensional dental implant planning system in the marketplace. The initial software, although revolutionary for the time, has undergone numerous technical advances. Some of the most recent modifications to the software include improved quality of the three-dimensional planning image, an expanded implant library to include more of the major implant manufacturers, a more accurate assessment of bone quality, abutment angulation specification, and an easier ordering system. All these improvements to the original software over the past 5 years allow for better predictability in outcome and make it a more user-friendly software system for the clinician [13,14].

The NobelGuide software system was developed in 2001 as a concept for virtual implant surgery, with the added benefit of fabrication of the final/temporary prosthesis before surgery. The software received US Food and Drug Administration (FDA) approval in 2005 with more than 1700 implants placed in the prelaunch phase of development. The overall benefits of this software system as compared with the Simplant software system rest mainly in its completeness in the diagnostic, treatment planning, surgical, and prosthetic phases of implant surgery. It is also advocated for use as a "flapless" surgical modality because of the purported accuracy of planning with the software program and predictability of the overall outcome.

The protocol for the NobelGuide software initially involves fabrication of a radiographic guide. The radiographic guide must be highly accurate and represent the patient's final prosthesis with regard to tooth positioning and occlusal relation. The radiographic guide is what permits the software to allow for surgical guide fabrication precisely and accurately and, eventually, a final prosthetic fabrication in a temporary or permanent form. The patient undergoes cone beam CT scanning, or conventional CT scanning, with the radiographic guide in place. The radiographic guide is also scanned separately from the patient. The two-scan technique is what allows the software program to overlap the images accurately, and thus provide a three-dimensional image of the patient with or without the radiographic guide in view. Once the cone beam CT images are downloaded and converted by the practitioner using the premium version of the software program, the treatment planning phase can be initiated. The software allows the practitioner to work with a three-dimensional model of the patient's jaw and prosthesis and with a radiographic image of the patient's jaw on the same computer screen (Fig. 3). As a result, the placement of implants can be controlled relative to the hard tissue architecture and emergence angle at the level of the prosthesis. Again, it is the accuracy of the radiographic guide that allows this to be possible, because it represents the final position of the future prosthetic dentition and occlusal relation. Once all the implant fixtures and anchor pins (used for improved soft tissue stabilization) have been designed by the practitioner using the software, a surgical guide is fabricated by the NobelGuide software program. After approving and placing the order for the surgical template and any surgical or prosthetic components, it takes approximately 1 week to have it delivered to the practitioner's office.

It is because of the high degree of accuracy with regard to fabrication of the radiographic guide and the cone beam imaging technology that NobelBiocare advocates the fabrication of a prosthetic solution for the patient before surgery. Although it is out of the realm of practice for an oral and maxillofacial surgeon to use the surgical template for fabrication of a prosthetic solution for the patient, it is, however, a beneficial adjunct to this particular implant surgical planning software.

The disadvantages of these systems is that they focus conceptually on the "ease" of implant surgery by advocating flapless surgical procedures, which entices the less surgically well-trained clinician to attempt advanced surgical procedures. The importance of a thorough and complete clinical diagnosis, based on proper surgical training, is somewhat overshadowed by sophisticated computer imaging techniques. Although flapless surgery can be a physiologic advantage to the patient from the standpoint of postoperative pain and swelling, it is not routinely the treatment of choice. It is often necessary to perform augmentation of hard or soft tissue simultaneously with implant placement. Experienced clinicians are better able to predict these scenarios, and thus plan for surgical alternatives before or during surgery. It is the inexperienced clinician who may inappropriately use these types of software systems with the intention of a flapless procedure that could result in the need for more advanced surgical intervention during surgery. Improper assessment of the patient's bony architecture and a resultant inaccurate decision-making process related to the lack of necessity for bone augmentation before surgery can result in a nonfavorable outcome for the patient. For instance, the possibility of soft tissue injuries as a result of improper diagnosis and implant placement design by the practitioner may be out of the scope of practice of the implant surgeon. It is therefore crucial that the use of implant surgical planning software provides the practitioner with supplemental rather than complete information in the overall treatment planning and surgical phases for his or her patient.

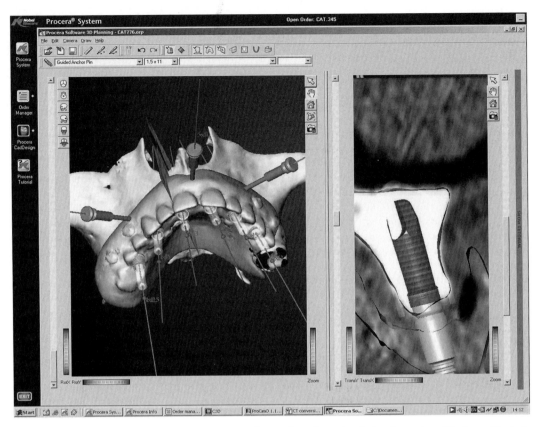

Fig. 3. On-screen image of the NobelBiocare Procera software three-dimensional planning system. The image illustrates the 3-dimensional implant planning phase with the prosthesis in place (*left side of image*) and the perpendicular radiographic image (*right side of image*), with an implant fixture placed ideally into the hard tissue architecture.

Computer technologies in orthognathic surgery

In the 1970s, planning for orthognathic surgery was through clinical examination, photographs, freehand surgical simulation based on cut-and-paste profile cephalometric tracings, and study model surgery [15,16]. The limitations of such planning techniques lay in the accuracy of the traced image because of radiographic distortion and human error. Also, the lack of predictability and visualization of the surgical outcome was a limiting factor for demonstration to the patient. In the 1980s, the integration of computer technologies in orthognathic surgery planning allowed for digitization of cephalometric tracing and simulation of surgical outcomes, permitting the patient to view and better appreciate the surgical treatment plan.

In 1986, Quick Ceph (San Diego, California) was developed by a German orthodontist, Gunther Blaseio, and introduced as one of the first orthognathic surgical planning software programs in the marketplace. Since then, numerous advancements in software design have led to the development and release of QC2000, which is marketed for orthodontists and oral and maxillofacial surgeons. This integrated system allows the clinician to capture and store high-resolution images, produce many predefined and customizable analyses, and generate growth forecasts and treatment simulations on line tracings and real images of patients. The curvatures in Quick Ceph outlines can be quickly and accurately edited by using control and anchor points, otherwise known as Bezier curves. Quick Ceph also allows the clinician to perform a model analysis to measure the arch length discrepancy (true and Moyers), the Bolton discrepancy, and the tooth size discrepancy. It comes with 10 lateral predefined analyses, 4 of which can quickly be redefined by any surgeon, resulting in thousands of user-defined analyses or combinations of them and a frontal analysis to determine if maxillary expansion is possible or if any asymmetries need to be corrected. It performs orthodontic and surgical movements in a single window.

The software also allows the practitioner to superimpose the initial, the growth phase, or the standard tracings during the treatment simulation to allow for realistic predictions. A flexible soft tissue analysis is included and allows the orientation of vertical reference lines to the natural head position (Spradley), to the Frankfurt, to the sella-nasion minus 7°, or to the glabella-nose minus 15° (Brons). The unique digital image enhancement function increases the quality of stored radiographs, making digitizing and tracing easier and more accurate. Quick Ceph images are compatible with all Macintosh and personal computer (PC)–based management software. They are also compatible with any digital radiographic machine that can export images in the Joint Photographic Experts Group (JPEG) format. As an added benefit to the private practitioner, expenses are minimized by eliminating film and the lack of necessity for employee time for handling and mounting pictures. The other advantage of QC2000 is that it allows for communication among professionals and between the clinician and his or her patients in a more efficient and effective manner.

Vistadent is another orthognathic software treatment planning program developed by Technocenter (GAC International, Birmingham, Alabama), which has the ability to locate orthodontic landmarks on cephalometric radiographs. It has the option of selecting 1 of 56 standard cephalometric analyses or creating a custom analysis allowing the operator to visualize treatment objectives and save multiple virtual outcomes by quickly creating Ricketts Visual Treatment Objective (VTO) using simple slider bars. It is also possible to perform virtual growth prediction and centric occlusion–centric relation corrections. Treatment simulation for surgery and orthodontics is possible from a single screen. This software system can also superimpose tracings done from any record series or virtual treatment, superimpose using landmarks or structures, and print superimpositions in single or segmented view. It is also compatible with all digital cameras and with most popular digital x-ray systems and digital model software packages.

Dentofacial Planner software (Dentofacial Planner Software Inc., Toronto, Ontario, Canada) was initially developed by an orthodontist as a computer-assisted instrument for diagnosis and planning for orthodontic treatment purposes only [17,18]. With further development of the system, including videocephalometric planning of the patient's treatment, the software was modified to allow for simulation of surgical operations. Traditionally, all imaging software programs use linear ratios for prediction of soft tissue changes after hard tissue movements, which means that they assume the soft tissue response is a fixed percentage of skeletal movement, regardless of skeletal change. Dentofacial Planner software uses nonlinear ratios with pattern recognition to predict soft tissue response. This approach is used to account for lip trap, incompetence, and mentalis strain more accurately. One of the limitations, however, is that although the ratio settings for other programs can be changed by the user, those for Dentofacial Planner software are hard-coded, and therefore cannot be customized [19].

Dolphin Imaging software developed by Dolphin Imaging and Management Solutions (Chatsworth, California) allows the clinician to use standard and customized analyses for treatment planning purposes. The lateral analyses include Ricketts, McNamara, Steiner (Tweed), Jarabak, Roth, Sassouni, McLaughlin, Bjork, Alexander (vari-simplex), Downs, Holdaway, Alabama, Burstone, Gerety, and many combinations and variations. Frontal analyses include Ricketts, Grummons, and Grummons simplified. Bolton and arch length discrepancy analyses are also possible using this software. The software is designed to allow for superimposition of cephalometric tracing over the patient's photograph and for superimpositioning of patient tracings at different time points with standard superimposition references (SN at sella, Frankfort at porion, Na-Pg at ANS-PNS, Na-Ba at CC, Na-Ba at Na, ANS-PNS at ANS, and Go-Me at Me). It also provides a special visual norm ("Profilogram") superimposition. The software calibrates radiographs for accuracy and automatically generates anatomic structures and profiles. It has easy image enhancements, such as zoom in/out, brightness, contrast, and sharpness, and can accurately align to Frankfort horizontal, horizontal plane (SN-7), or the natural head position. The treatment simulation allows the clinician to plan, diagnose, and present cases from the lateral view. It can be used for orthodontics and surgical applications. Specifically from a surgery standpoint, simulation of LeFort osteotomies, bilateral sagittal split osteotomy (BSSO), multiple jaw surgery, and genioplasty is easily visualized. Cosmetic rhinoplasty procedures and zygomatic implants can also be simulated on this software with image touch-up and morphing tools. It is an easy tool of communication with referring clinicians and patients. It is also network-ready for image access anywhere in the office, and it exports images to any standard file format. It integrates with all digital radiographic systems.

Clearly, numerous software programs for cephalometric analysis, diagnosis, growth prediction, surgical planning, and prediction are available in the marketplace [20]. The clinician should question the accuracy with which these programs predict the actual outcome of treatment, however. Many clinicians have conducted research evaluating the accuracy of orthognathic surgical prediction based on cephalometric programs. As is the case with manual cephalometric tracing, the computerized tracing is also prone to errors. It is the responsibility of the practitioner to recognize these limitations so that they can be minimized and accounted for when planning orthognathic surgical procedures. Keeping up to date with the rapidly evolving world of hardware and software digitization programs has become an additional aspect of literature review for the clinician [19]. Anecdotal evidence has shown that prediction is less accurate when major vertical changes in jaw position are performed [19]. In the line drawings era, Dentofacial Planner was found to be accurate in predicting the nose and chin position, but a significant difference in lip predictions was noted [21–23]. Schultes and colleagues [24] studied the soft tissue prediction in the vertical plane of 25 patients with mandibular retrognathia with Dentofacial Planner and found that the nose and the chin position were accurate, whereas the highest degree of error occurred in the submental area.

Loh and colleagues [25] conducted a retrospective study to analyze the accuracy and reliability of predictions generated in 28 heterogeneous patients treated with orthognathic surgery by comparing Quick Ceph Image Pro predictions with postsurgical lateral cephalographs. They found that 10 of the 14 parameters measured in this study had no significant differences between the predicted and actual postsurgical hard tissue landmarks. The 4 parameters that showed statistically significant differences were ANB ($P = .008$), FMA ($P = .001$), SN-Mx1 ($P = .03$), and Wit's analysis ($P = .0001$). Although these values were statistically significant, 3 of the 4 parameters (ANB, FMA, and SN-Mx1) showed a maximal difference of 3.2°, which was clinically insignificant. The magnitude of these differences was less than the errors reported with manual cephalometric tracing [25]. Wit's analysis was the only parameter that showed statistical and clinical significant differences, with the greatest being operator variability [25]. This finding is not surprising, given that the Wit's value involves determination of the functional occlusal plane, which, in turn, relies on the accurate identification of six landmarks. As such, even if the Wit's value may be valid for diagnosis, it is clearly not reliable for orthognathic surgery planning [19]. In 1997, Aharon and colleagues [26] compared Dentofacial Planner and Quick Ceph Image software and found that both programs performed well in simulating single-jaw and double-jaw operations. With Quick Ceph Image, only the predicted value of the horizontal position of the upper lip differed significantly from the actual postsurgical outcome. With Dentofacial Planner, the positions of the lower lip and soft tissue menton were significantly different [26].

In 2000, Curtis and colleagues [27] evaluated Orthognathic Treatment Planner (GAC International, Birmingham, Alabama), a predecessor of Vistadent. The predicted position of the upper lip was accurate at 80%, but that of the lower lip was less than 50% accurate. In 2003, Lu and colleagues [28] evaluated the accuracy of the outcome in soft tissue prediction by using Dolphin Imaging system software (version 6) after bimaxillary orthognathic surgery. In the 30 patients who underwent combined Wassmund and Kole procedures with an optional genioplasty to correct bimaxillary protrusion, they found that the nasal tip, soft tissue A point, and upper lip presented the least amount of predicted errors in the sagittal plane [28]. Contrary to the findings with the nasal tip, the lower lip prediction was the least accurate and was mostly positioned more anterior to the actual position. The predictions were generally more accurate in the vertical plane as opposed to the sagittal plane. There was no statistical significance between the predictions of the groups with or without genioplasty [28].

Smith and colleagues [19] chose 10 difficult test cases with vertical discrepancies and "retreated" them using the actual surgical changes to investigate perceived differences in the ability of current software to simulate the actual outcome of orthognathic surgery. They evaluated five programs—Dentofacial Planner Plus, Dolphin Imaging, Orthoplan (Orthographics Inc., Salt Lake City, Utah), Quick Ceph Image, and Vistadent—by using the default result and a refined result created with each program's enhancement tools. Three panels consisting of orthodontists, oral maxillofacial surgeons, and laypersons judged the default images and the retouched simulations by ranking the simulations in side-by-side comparisons and by rating each simulation relative to the actual outcome on a six-point scale. Dentofacial Planner Plus was judged the best default simulation software. It also scored best when the retouched images were compared with Dolphin Imaging and Quick Ceph. Retouching had little impact on the scores for the other programs. What do these findings mean for the practitioner with regard to choosing the right imaging software? The decision depends on multiple factors. Accuracy in predictability, ease of use, cost, and compatibility with other practice management tools are all important considerations. Concerns with operating system compatibility, practice management integration, and staff training warrant the need for excellent customer service and timely and efficient technical support by the software distributors.

Computer technologies in stereolithographic modeling

What is stereolithographic biomodeling? It is a modern technology that transforms three-dimensional CT data into solid plastic replicas of anatomic structures (biomodels) [29–35]. The possibility of generating a three-dimensional model from CT scans was first mentioned in 1980, and reconstruction of the first craniofacial foam model took place in 1987 [36]. The availability of this type of technology allows for the fabrication of a life-sized model of deformed, fractured, or otherwise altered craniofacial structures, permitting the surgeon to observe directly and plan the necessary surgical intervention before surgery. Fig. 4 represents an example of a stereolithographic reconstruction of a patient with bilateral condylar resorption causing a significant anterior open bite. Although a highly accurate model can be constructed using this technology, the main limitation is the high cost to the patient and practitioner, making it a secondary choice for most surgeons.

The accuracy of stereolithography in planning craniofacial bone replacement was studied by Chang and colleagues [37]. The mean error found was less than 2 mm, representing a percentage error of 5%. This error is consistent with other studies, which show an accuracy ranging between 0.6% and 6.0% [37]. They found that the greatest error occurred in the midface, wherein the thinness and complexity of the bone are prone to misreads in the data acquisition phase during the initial scan. They recommend obtaining an amount of tissue at least 1 cm greater than that of predicted value to account for errors in prediction [37].

Other applications of stereolithographic biomodeling are in endosseous dental implant surgical planning, wherein an accurate knowledge of anatomic structures is important, and in severe dentofacial deformities for planning orthognathic surgery [38]. Gateno and colleagues [39] used stereolithography to examine the in vitro accuracy of distraction osteogenesis of the mandible that involved a planning process and a surgical technique. There was an excellent correlation between the predicted and actual measurements for the X, Y, and Z axes. Biomodeling has become a highly reliable technology during the past few years and is being used routinely in complicated craniofacial surgery.

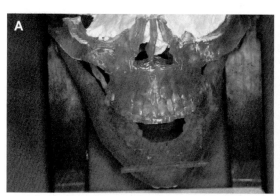
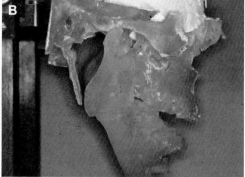

Fig. 4. Stereolithographic models in the frontal (A) and lateral (B) views representing a patient with bilateral condylar resorption resulting in a significant anterior open bite.

Some of the limitations associated with stereolithographic biomodeling include precision of details in the reconstructed models, the artifacts of CT scanning, the representation of bone structures without contact with surrounding bone structures, postproduction resin shrinkage of the models, increased exposure to radiation, and the cost of stereolithographic models [36]. Stereolithography has potential applications in routine use for dentoalveolar reconstruction and implant surgery and as a patient educational tool. For the present, because of the cost and increased exposure to radiation, this technique is limited to planning complex craniofacial reconstructions, significant maxillofacial asymmetries, and distraction osteogenesis. In these cases, the benefits outweigh the risks. Further studies are needed to simulate the soft tissue changes incurred by hard tissue manipulation in stereolithography. As a result, the introduction of a specific treatment to a local anatomic region can better be assessed three dimensionally in a regional environment.

Summary

The integration of computer technology in the practice of oral and maxillofacial surgery has been a steady and relatively unencumbered process. Not all aspects of computer technology are favorable, and most of the limitations exist because of the rapidity of developing these software programs and the limited scientific research before their release. Also, the learning curve for most software programs and their high cost have been a hindrance to the wide acceptance of such technologies in established oral and maxillofacial surgery practices. Computer technology does seem to be quickly gaining favor with the new generation of surgeons being trained in our specialty, however. The need for such technologies is clear, and the advantages that they present are numerous. Yet, the cost factor and limited availability of intensive training programs for these technologies are likely to make overall acceptance and use a slow process. It is therefore the responsibility of the developers of these new technologies to play an integral part not only in the development and sales aspect but, more importantly, in the funding of controlled experimental studies to evaluate and compare the pros and cons of their products. The clinician's responsibility, conversely, is to be well informed of the currently available software programs and to become more educated regarding their potential uses, limitations, and overall benefits to the practice of oral and maxillofacial surgery.

References

[1] White SC, Heslop EW, Hollender LG, et al. American Academy of Oral and Maxillofacial Radiology, ad hoc Committee on Parameters of Care. Parameters of radiologic care: an official report of the American Academy of Oral and Maxillofacial Radiology. Oral Surg Oral Med Oral Pathol Oral Radiol Endod 2001;91(5):498–511.

[2] Scarfe WC, Farman AG, Sukovic P. Clinical applications of cone-beam computer tomography in dental practice. J Can Dent Assoc 2006;72(1):75–80.

[3] Sukovic P. Cone beam computed tomography in craniofacial imaging. Orthod Craniofac Res 2003; 6(Suppl 1):31–6.

[4] Hashimoto K, Arai Y, Iwai K, et al. A comparison of a new limited cone beam computed tomography machine for dental use with a multidetector row helical CT machine. Oral Surg Oral Med Oral Pathol Oral Radiol Endod 2004;95:371–7.

[5] Ito K, Gomi Y, Sato S, et al. Clinical application of a new compact CT system to assess 3-D images for the preoperative treatment planning of implants in the posterior mandible. A case report. Clin Oral Implants Res 2001;12:539–42.

[6] Nakagawa Y, Kobayashi K, Ishii H, et al. Preoperative application of limited cone beam computerized tomography as an assessment tool before minor oral surgery. Int J Oral Maxillofac Surg 2002;32:322–7.

[7] Kobayashi K, Shimoda S, Nakagawa Y, et al. Accuracy in measurement of distance using limited cone-beam computed tomography. Int J Oral Maxillofac Implants 2004;19:228–31.

[8] Ludlow JB, Davies-Ludlow LE, Brooks SL, et al. Dosimetry of 3 CBCT devices for oral and maxillofacial radiology: CB Mercuray, NewTom 3G, and i-CAT. Dentomaxillofac Radiol 2006;35:219–26. Erratum in Dentomaxillofac Radiol 2006;35:392.

[9] Hirsch E, Graf H-L, Hemprich A. Comparative investigation of image quality of three different X-ray procedures. Dentomaxillofac Radiol 2003;32: 201–11.

[10] Mah JK, Danforth RA, Bumann A, et al. Radiation absorbed in maxillofacial imaging with a new dental computed tomography device. Oral Surg Oral Med Oral Pathol Oral Radiol Endod 2003;96:508–13.

[11] Ngan DC, Kharbanda OP, Geenty JP, et al. Comparison of radiation levels from computed tomography and conventional dental radiographs. Aust Orthod J 2003;19:67–75.

[12] Sarment DP, Sukovic P, Clinthorne N. Accuracy of implant placement with a stereolithographic surgical guide. Int J Oral Maxillofac Implants 2003;18:571–7.

[13] Al-Faraje L. The benefits of computer-guided implantology and Surgi-guides in treating patients with advanced alveolar bone resorption. Materialise Headlines 2004;4:3–5. Available at: http://www.materialise.com/materialise/view/en/473249-Materialise+Headlines.html.

[14] Mandelaris GA, Rosenfeld AL. Is the technology trustworthy? Clinical transition from bone to tooth supported surgi-guides. Materialize Headlines 2005; 3:2–3. Available at: http://www.materialise.com/_marketing_/HEADLINES/PDF/Headlines3_2005_EU.pdf.

[15] Loh S, Yow M. Computer prediction of hard tissue profiles in orthognathic surgery. Int J Adult Orthodon Orthognath Surg 2002;17:342–7.

[16] Vig KD, Ellis E. Diagnosis and treatment planning for the surgical-orthodontic patient. Dent Clin North Am 1990;34:361–84.

[17] Csaszar GR, Bruker-Csaszar B, Niederdellmann H. Prediction of soft tissue profiles in orthodontic surgery with the Dentofacial Planner. Int J Adult Orthodon Orthognath Surg 1999;14:285–90.

[18] Seeholzer H, Walker R. Orthodontic and oral surgical treatment planning by computer, for example, the Dentofacial Planners. Quintessenz 1991;42:59–67.

[19] Smith JD, Thomas P, Proffit WR. A comparison of current prediction imaging programs. Am J Orthod Dentofacial Orthop 2004;125:527–36.

[20] Ricketts RM, Bench R, Hilgers JJ, et al. An overview of computerized cephalometrics. Am J Orthod 1972; 61:1–28.

[21] Konstiantos KA, O'Reilly MT, Close J. The validity of the prediction of soft tissue profile changes after Le Fort I osteotomy using Dentofacial Planner (computer software). Am J Orthod Dentofacial Orthop 1994;105:241–9.

[22] Kolokitha OE, Athanasiou AE, Tuncay OC. Validity of computerized predictions of dentoskeletal and soft tissue profile changes after mandibular setback and maxillary impaction osteotomies. Int J Adult Orthodon Orthognath Surg 1996;11:137–54.

[23] Eales EA, Newton C, Jones ML, et al. The accuracy of computerized prediction of the soft tissue profile—a study of 25 patients treated by means of the Le Fort I osteotomy. Int J Adult Orthodon Orthognath Surg 1994;9:141–52.

[24] Schultes G, Gaggl A, Karcher H. Accuracy of cephalometric and video imaging program Dentofacial Planner Plus in orthognathic surgical planning. Comput Aided Surg 1998;3:108–14.

[25] Loh S, Heng K, Ward-Booth P, et al. A radiographic analysis of computer prediction in conjunction with orthognathic surgery. Int J Oral Maxillofac Surg 2001;30:259–63.

[26] Aharon PA, Eisig S, Cisneros GJ. Surgical prediction reliability—a comparison of two computer software systems. Int J Adult Orthodon Orthognath Surg 1997;12:65–78.

[27] Curtis TJ, Casko JS, Jakobsen JR, et al. Accuracy of a computerized method of predicting soft-tissue changes from orthognathic surgery. J Clin Orthod 2000;34:524–30.

[28] Lu CH, Ko E, Huang CS. The accuracy of video imaging prediction in soft tissue outcome after bimaxillary orthognathic surgery. J Oral Maxillofac Surg 2003;61:333–42.

[29] Xia J, Ip HHS, Samman N, et al. Computer-assisted three-dimensional surgical planning and simulation: 3D virtual osteotomy. Int J Oral Maxillofac Surg 2000;29:11–7.

[30] Xia J, Samman N, Yeung RWK, et al. Three-dimensional virtual reality surgical planning and simulation workbench for orthognathic surgery. Int J Adult Orthodon Orthognath Surg 2000;15:265–82.

[31] Bill JS, Reuther JF, Dittman W, et al. Stereolithography in oral and maxillofacial operation planning. Int J Oral Maxillofac Surg 1995;24:98–103.

[32] D'Urso PS, Barker TM, Earwaker WJ, et al. Stereolithographic biomodeling in cranio-maxillofacial surgery: a prospective trial. J Craniomaxillofac Surg 1999;27:30–7.

[33] Erickson DM, Chance D, Schmitt S, et al. An opinion survey of reported benefits from the use of stereolithographic models. J Oral Maxillofac Surg 1999;57:1041–3.

[34] Kermer C, Rasse M, Lagogiannis G, et al. Color stereolithography for planning complex maxillofacial tumor surgery. J Craniomaxillofac Surg 1998; 26:360–2.

[35] Kragslov J, Sindet-Pedersen S, Gyldensted C, et al. A comparison of three-dimensional computed tomography scans and stereolithographic models for evaluation of craniofacial anomalies. J Oral Maxillofac Surg 1996;54:402–11.

[36] Sailer HF, Haers PE, Zollikofer CPE, et al. The value of stereolithographic models for preoperative diagnosis of craniofacial deformities and planning of surgical corrections. Int J Oral Maxillofac Surg 1998;27:327–33.

[37] Chang PSH, Parker TH, Patrick CW, et al. The accuracy of stereolithography in planning craniofacial bone replacement. J Craniofac Surg 2003;14:164–70.

[38] Arvier JF, Barker TM, Yau YY, et al. Maxillofacial biomodeling. Br J Oral Maxillofac Surg 1994;32:276–83.

[39] Gateno J, Teichgraeber JF, Messersmith ML. An in vitro study of the accuracy of a new protocol for planning distraction osteogenesis of the mandible. J Oral Maxillofac Surg 2000;58:985–90.

Web Marketing for Oral and Maxillofacial Surgeons

Chad Brandt, BA[a,b,c]

[a]Active Internet Solutions, Chicago, IL, USA
[b]National Foundation for Celiac Awareness, Ambler, PA, USA
[c]The University of Chicago Graduate School of Business, Chicago, IL, USA

Marketing is important to any business. Whether you intend attract new customers, keep existing clients, or expand into new areas, marketing will play an important role. Most small businesses have very limited time and resources for marketing, so it is crucial that the investment receives a significant return. Advertising your business via the internet is a great way to stretch marketing dollars and have the information about your doctors, practice, and services available 24 hours a day. When your practice closes for the day, the Web site continues work by providing customer support, practice details, and critical information needed by patients, referring doctors, health care providers, and potential clients.

In the course of this chapter, we explain why your practice needs a Web site, how you go about setting up a site, and what to expect during the process. For those who know very little regarding the internet and Web publishing, beyond e-mail, browsing the Web, and online shopping, this can be a very intimidating process. With a brief overview, you will be ready to set up your practice's first Web site (Fig. 1) and begin Web marketing with confidence.

Why should my practice have a Web site?

The benefits of having a Web site are too numerous to count. A Web site provides information about your practice 24 hours a day, 7 days a week.

Benefits

24-hour customer service

Think of the Web site as an employee, providing great customer service to those looking for information regarding your practice. This employee works nonstop and can be extremely effective. The information provided consists of contact information including phone numbers and address locations, practice e-mail address, patient forms, hours of operation, maps and directions, practice history, service offerings and descriptions, doctor biographies, and frequently asked questions (FAQ). An FAQ section can take some unnecessary burden off of your front desk staff. Photos and biographies of doctors and staff can be posted to provide a personal connection for patients before stepping foot into the office [1]. Office photos can be posted to showcase your state-of-the-art practice and improve patient familiarity. Patients will become less apprehensive regarding their visit if they know what to expect. Providing information about services and procedures can help differentiate your practice from competitors. Many new patients will seek out your Web site first, educate themselves on your services, and save you and your staff the trouble of explaining these services at length. This may save time during first consultations with patients. Furthermore, posting patient documentation to be downloaded and filled out before visit is a great way to add efficiency to the check-in process. Why force visitors to fill out paperwork in your office (Fig. 2)? Provide as much information to new patients up front on the Web site and reduce the time that the patient needs to be at the office. This is good for both the patient and the practice.

Flexibility

A Web site is an extremely flexible medium as opposed to print. It may take several hours to update your Web site with new contact information or a change in your service offerings, but your entire line of brochures would need to be

E-mail address: hello@chadbrandt.com

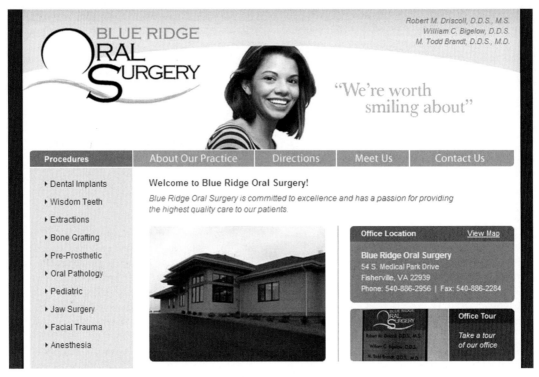

Fig. 1. Blue Ridge Oral Surgery Homepage. (*Courtesy of* Blue Ridge Oral Surgery, Fishersville, VA; with permission.)

redesigned and reprinted. This change to print material can be time consuming and costly. Investing more time and effort into your Web site will allow you to adapt more quickly and provide up-to-date information to your patients, prospects, and referring doctors.

Branding

A well-designed Web site can improve and evolve the professional brand of your practice [2]. Connect your offline brand (ie, print materials or office décor) to your online brand. A Web site address can be listed on all marketing materials,

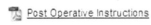
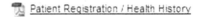

Fig. 2. Download important forms directly from the homepage. (*Courtesy of* Blue Ridge Oral Surgery, Fishersville, VA; with permission.)

such as business cards, brochures, after-visit bags, pens, notepads, and nail files. This Web address provides a living extension to those marketing materials and gives customers a place to visit at anytime to learn more about your practice. Whereas the print materials may remain static to reduce costs, the Web site can be updated frequently and provide the latest, most accurate information for your audience.

Communication, beyond patients

A Web site is an excellent method of communication for your practice's entire audience [3]. This may include, beyond existing patients, referring doctors or dentists, hospitals, health care providers, staff members, parents and guardians of young patients, dental and oral surgery associations, your local community, and so on. It is also a great way to establish your doctors in the medical or dental community by providing updated biographies (Fig. 3), Curricula vitae, research, publications, and other accomplishments. It is an excellent networking tool.

A Web site will also come with e-mail addresses for your practice. This is another way for you to keep connected with your patients and an additional method to extend the brand of your practice. A phone number says nothing about the business for which it is attached. An e-mail address, *office@youroralsurgerypractice.com* provides a direct link between the patient and your staff and your practice. It's easy for a patient to remember and a quick way to communicate with your office.

Search engine availability

It is important to have your practice available on the Web for new patients to find when searching the Web for oral surgeons in their area [4]. Creating a Web site and having it listed with search engines is very important. At the very least, your Web site should be listed in results

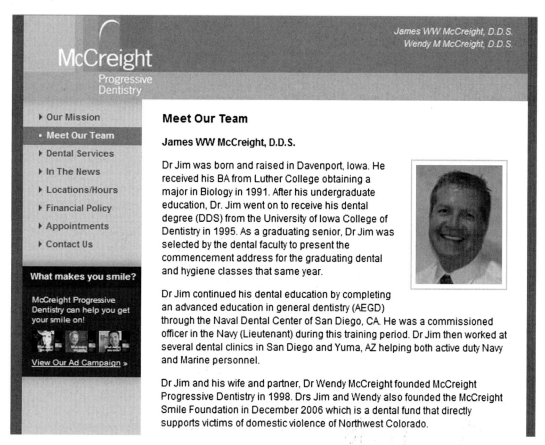

Fig. 3. Sample biography from McCreight Progressive Dentistry (*mccreightsmiles.com*). (*Courtesy of* McCreight Progressive Dentistry, Steamboat Springs, CO; with permission.)

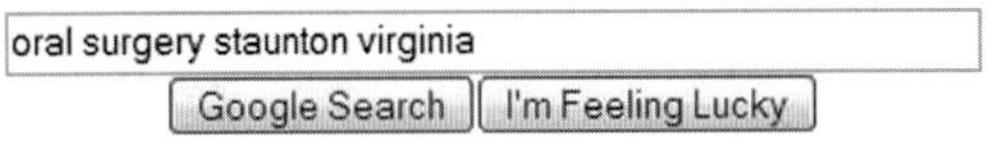

Fig. 4. Google search for "oral surgery" plus location. (*Courtesy of* Google, Inc., Mountain View, CA; with permission.)

when a potential client searches for your practice name, the names of your doctors, and possibly the combination of the words "oral surgery" and the county, city, or state of your practice (Fig. 4).

Keeping in touch

As your Web site evolves, news stories can be posted (perhaps on a monthly or weekly basis) regarding your office/staff/doctors, regarding new developments in oral surgery, your practice, or changes in services. Many practices will improve ongoing communication with patients that may not visit the office frequently. The Web site, coupled with e-mail newsletters or a regular mailing, will help keep the lines of communication open and hopefully increase repeat business and patient referrals.

What are the costs?

A practice Web site consists of a reasonable short-term investment, small monthly maintenance charges, and large long-term gain.

Cost breakdown

Domain name "rental" ($8-35 per year)

This secures your practice's presence on the Web with www.yourpracticename.com [5]. Domain rental does not cover Web site or e-mail hosting, that's extra. Domain names are acquired through Registrars. This is usually separate from your Web hosting company. Although, many Web hosting companies will offer this as an added value service. Typically, it is best to choose a domain registrar the main focus of which is registering domain names. A company like GoDaddy (Fig. 5) offers domains on an average of $8.99 per year. This is a fantastic price that comes with excellent service. The same domain name can cost $35 at a company like Network Solutions. There is no difference in registration between these 2 companies—Disclaimer: Choose a well-established, proven company like GoDaddy for registrations to ensure good service and a pleasant experience. Lastly, your Web design firm may offer to maintain your domain name registration for a small fee. This is a great idea

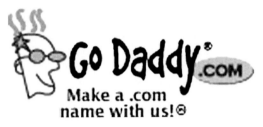

Fig. 5. GoDaddy logo. (*Courtesy of* GoDaddy.com, Inc., Scottsdale, AZ; with permission.)

to reduce the hassle of registering and renewing yourself year to year. A typical Web design firm will maintain dozens of domain names and will be best suited to keep this information current and active (Fig. 6).

Site design and build ($1500-$10,000+)

You will need to choose a design/marketing firm or Web consultant to produce the Web site design and build out the entire site. Depending on the size, features, and complexity of your Web site, this one-time fee can range between $1500 and $10,000 or higher. The higher price will usually include some sort of online content management system in which you or your staff can update the site yourself. The higher price may also cover multimedia interactive Web sites that use technologies such as flash or video. For the average oral surgeon, this level of interactivity is unnecessary. A static Web site, which provides relevant text-based content for visitors while also being visually appealing, will be more than suitable for effective marketing purposes. A good-quality Web site, on average, will cost between $3000 and $5000. This price pays for a high level of expertise and proficiency in graphic design, Web design, and Web project management. The lower price, around $1500, will most likely be offered by a Web developer who can code and design the Web site without additional assistance. In these cases, you will have a working Web site, but you will not pay for experience, expertise, or a Web site that will function well for search

Fig. 6. Register.com logo. (*Courtesy of* Register.com, Inc., New York, NY; with permission.)

engines and future compatibility of Web browsers, nor will it provide a professional look for your business. The rule of "get what you pay for" certainly applies in Web site design and production. Best practice: Stay somewhere around the middle range for Web design and site development.

You will need to determine how much your marketing firm will control in terms of your brand. Do you have an existing marketing presence with a company logo, business cards, brochure, and other print materials? Is that brand continued through your office? If so, that existing information will save you time and money when developing your Web site. Expect to pay more if you approach a design/marketing firm with both the development of your office brand as well as a functional Web site.

Web site and e-mail hosting ($30-$100 per month)

Hosting refers to placing your Web site files (graphics, photos, text, documents) on a server. That server computer hosts your Web site files and makes them available on the internet via an Internet Protocol (IP) address (example: 00.000.00.00). When your site goes live or is "launched," your domain name is pointed to this IP address. The practice's domain name is now connected to the hosting server (Fig. 7). Web site hosting can cost between $30 and $100+ per month. Again, the higher side may cover a site that has a content management system or high-end video and graphics. This monthly hosting fee may also include ongoing maintenance. For example, a typical Web design firm may host for $50 per month and include several hours of free Web site updates. If a Web firm

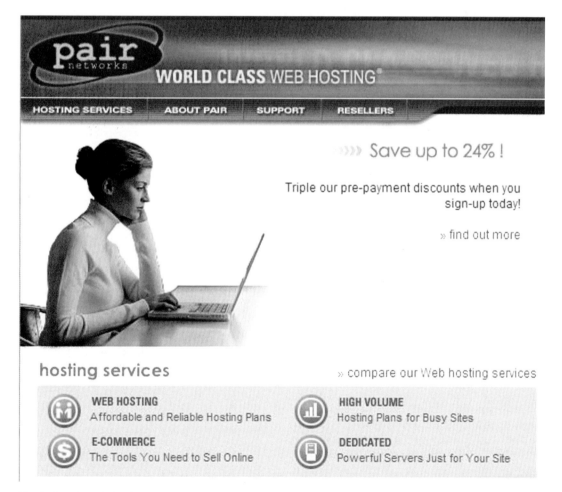

Fig. 7. Sample Web hosting company site, pair networks (*pair.com*). (*Courtesy of* pair Networks, Pittsburgh, PA; with permission.)

charges $75 per hour for updates, including monthly maintenance with hosting, this is a great deal. The low end of the hosting scale will require someone from your office to manage hosting with an online service. They will need to maintain the relationship with the hosting company and become familiar with the technology. It is best to pay a little more for your Web design firm to host your Web site or recommend a provider that can do so without requiring the client to have technical experience.

E-mail hosting should never be an extra cost. It should be included with all hosting packages. Also, you should not be limited by the number of e-mail accounts. Most hosting plans offer unlimited e-mail accounts with no additional cost.

Costs for hosting can increase with higher Web site traffic and serving large files to more visitors. Also, costs for hosting can change based on the selected server technologies. Open source servers (Linux) will be cheaper than a server running Microsoft Windows. For most practices with very basic Web sites and no dynamic functionality, open source servers will be adequate.

Web site maintenance (hourly rate)

Ongoing fees for your Web site may include hourly Web site maintenance to update content, photos, staff members, doctor bios, and other information. This should be included in the hosting contract and paid hourly after a certain number of hours per month. These services may range from $30 to $75 per hour. Updating text on a Web site is quicker and easier than updating photos and graphics. Also, keep in mind that a change to your Web site may affect more than a single page. It is good practice to ask your consulting firm or Web developer to provide a time estimate for the updates. It is also good to group your updates in a batch so they can be accomplished together. This will reduce time and costs.

Other potential costs

Additional costs for your Web site project may include advanced search engine optimization, site optimization to make your site run faster, Web site maintenance, and Web applications such as online forms, traffic analysis, and e-mail campaigns.

Some practices may need only updates to their existing Web sites to improve design, content, and search engine rankings. Those practices can expect to pay an hourly rate for updates from $30 to $75/per hour or a flat rate that may be a little less than a from-scratch Web design project. If content and design exist and can be salvaged, a code redesign (the structure beneath your Web site) can be accomplished for around $1500. This is a great way to improve your Web site for visitors and search engines. The rest of the services listed above may not be necessary for the average oral surgery practice. E-mail campaigns can be handled by internal staff or a company that specializes in this type of marketing for oral surgeons.

Traffic analysis can be provided to you cheaply using a service like Google Analytics, Stat Monitor, or Hitbox.

If you want clients to fill out patient forms online and submit the information with the click of a button, expect to pay a Web application developer $50 to $100+ per hour to build this type of functionality. Posting forms as PDFs for patient download is a great alternative and requires no advanced programming.

How do I build a site for my practice? Where do I start?

Choose a domain name

Start with the name of your practice and choose a domain name that's easy to type and not too long. Remember, this domain name will be typed into Web browsers and most likely used for your e-mail addresses. Although an abbreviation may be easy to remember and quick to type, it is best to choose a name that provides some information about your practice. For example, bros.com, although short and easy to type, may not be as effective as blueridgeoralsurgery.com. Keep in mind, the longer domain name contains very simple words so the length does not present much difficulty for visitors. Lastly, make sure your domain is available and then register the domain. You can check the availability by typing the domain into a browser and see if any results come up. From there, you can enter the domain name into a registrar's site, such as GoDaddy or Network Solutions, to see if it's available. Once an available name is found, register the domain through an online service or have your Web design firm take care of it for you.

Determine the project lead

Determine the project lead or team from your office who will manage the Web site development and ongoing Web marketing initiative. This person or team should have enough time to devote to this type of project. This is an important part of your marketing strategy and requires time to develop. Make sure your team is not too large. Many times, a project team will bring their own likes and dislikes regarding Web sites to this project. This is not about individual preferences of the doctors and staff. This is about communicating in the best way possible to your patients and additional audience as well as reinforcing your brand. Provide information simply and quickly to visitors and stay true to the image of your business.

Develop site content

Start writing your content and outline pages for your site. This can start with existing materials such as a brochure. Outline the site with top-level pages such as home, mission statement, services, doctors, staff, practice history, about us, frequently asked questions, office locations, and contact us. Once you have this simple outline, produce a few paragraphs of content for each of the pages. For the homepage, provide teasers to the most important information and link to important pages within the Web site. The outline will also serve as the start of the navigation for your Web site. Providing this information to your marketing firm or Web consultant early in the design process will be extremely beneficial and will save time and money. It is much easier for a graphic designer to produce the look and feel of your site after reading your site content.

Gather information for design firm

Write down ideas for how you want to market your business online. What sites do you like? What don't you like? Why? Produce a list of 5 sample Web sites in your business category to show examples of what you would like to incorporate into your site. Your comments can be as simple as: The navigation for this site is simple and intuitive; the content for these pages is great; the color scheme works well for their brand; the design of this site is great overall. Refrain from gathering sample sites like *yahoo.com*, *cnn.com*, or your favorite blog or shopping site. Find good, sample Web sites within the areas of oral surgery or medicine. These will be most helpful for your consulting firm during art direction and design phases.

In addition to these examples, collect digital assets such as company logo, print materials including business cards and letterhead, and photos of staff members, doctors, and your offices. It may be beneficial to have some of these photos taken professionally. These deliverables along with your outline, site content, and list of example sites will provide a perfect foundation to begin working with a Web consultant or design/marketing firm. In addition, take the time to write a quick paragraph regarding the mission for the Web site. What do you want it to do for your practice, and how would you like it to be used. I encourage clients to write "stories" for how they envision their Web site will be used. A brief story is sometimes more effective in communicating a message than writing a list of needed feature requirements.

Find and select a Web design firm

Research and contact Web design firms, Web marketing companies, or Web consultants in your area and ask them to provide an estimate for Web site design, site production, Web hosting, site maintenance, and other services. Ask for recommendations from colleagues or businesses in your area. Meet or speak briefly with leads at various firms, state your needs briefly, and ask for a written estimate (via e-mail is efficient). After you have compiled a list of design firms and consultants, review their estimates, peruse sample sites, and ask follow-up questions if certain services, deliverables, or costs are unclear.

Find a Web design firm that shares this view and will partner with your to make sure your customers receive the best possible online experience. Develop a good working relationship with your Web marketing firm and work toward a mutual goal.

Understand your deliverables from the Web design firm. A good firm will ask the client to provide content, digital assets (listed above), and ideas for the Web site before starting the design process. With this information, the design firm can develop a site specifically for your practice. Be wary of a firm that does not require this information and does not initiate a "discovery" before starting designs. Without this discovery, your site will be just another cookie cutter Web site. It will not be personal or specific to your business and brand. Typically, large Web site providers that also provide business services such as oral surgery software, automation, or online patient appointments, will see Web sites as a secondary service. They will most likely provide a cookie cutter site and not worry about the details of your practice. A site like this will not benefit your brand or the personality of your practice.

Once an estimate is approved and a design firm chosen, ask the firm or consultant to provide a written contract for the project. The contract should include a breakdown of costs for all portions of the project including discovery, graphic design, site production, testing, and launch. The contract should specify how many designs you will receive for the Web site and how much additional design work will cost after those included designs or base number of hours. A timeline and proposed launch date should be stated in the contract. Also, the contract should address legal considerations such as ownership of digital assets and responsibility of various parties. You should not select a vendor that does not provide a contract. This can cause problems for both parties.

Create the site

After a contract is approved and signed, you can begin working with the design firm. They should perform their discovery and collect your assets and input for the project. From there, they can begin developing visual ideas and recommendations for the site layout and architecture.

Make sure your design firm keeps you informed during the development process. Ask to review design work. Depending on how much you have paid, the design firm will be able to show you a few ideas for the design of your site. Typically, a design will be created for the homepage and an interior page of the site (Fig. 8). Provide feedback and then receive another iteration during the design process. Your marketing firm will most likely set a limit on the iterations during the design process. Be aware of these limits and make sure your feedback is heard and incorporated into

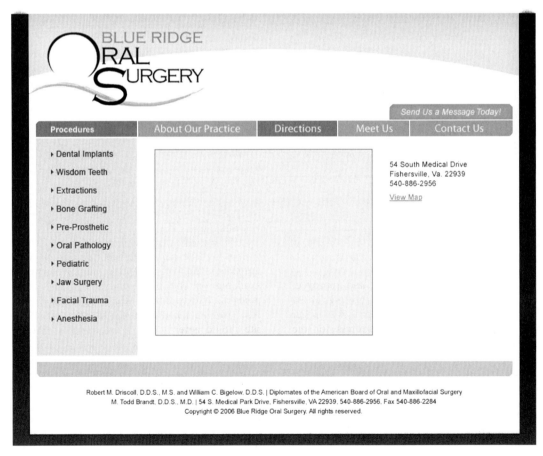

Fig. 8. Sample page design for *blueridgeoralsurgery.com*. (*Courtesy of* Blue Ridge Oral Surgery, Fishersville, VA; with permission.)

the design. By paying a higher price for the design, you most likely will receive better quality from the start.

Once the design is approved, the building process or site production will begin. This is where the design firm takes the approved mock-ups or pages (homepage and interior template) and incorporates your content and site hierarchy to produce clickable pages and navigation. You will start to see your ideas develop into a working Web site. At this stage, you should provide feedback per page regarding content changes, small layout issues, and adding photos to enhance certain pages. Adding pages at this stage should not be a major issue. Once a single page template is created, it is not difficult to add new pages. Be wary of design firms that charge per additional page.

Review

At this point, the Web site should be nearly complete. Make sure a few people on staff review every page of the site for accuracy.

Before launch, ask the design firm to confirm that the site is ready for search engine submissions including meta tags, page titles, and proper headlines incorporating keywords. Your design firm should ask for a list of relevant keywords and a description for search engine optimization. Also ask that your site have available traffic analysis before launch. This should be included in your hosting package.

Test your Web site on multiple platforms and browsers. Make sure it works and appears the same on all operating systems and browsers. If you have forms or documents on your site, make sure each of those works properly.

Launch your Web site

The site is complete, reviewed, and approved. The Web firm should have secured hosting for the Web site and is ready to flip the switch to connect your domain name to the IP address for the hosting server. The launch process should take no more than a day to complete. Test again after launch and make sure your site is available at your domain name.

After several weeks, your site should become available on search engines. This occurs as long as your Web firm takes appropriate steps to submit your site to the large search engines: *yahoo.com*, *msn.com*, and *google.com*. It is not necessary to pay extra for a submission service. Your Webmaster can also add a Google sitemap to ensure that your site is spidered quickly, and the content is available for searches. Keep reading for more ways to improve search engine ranking and site availability.

The site is done, now what?

Check or update your marketing materials

Make sure your Web address is listed on all marketing materials. Also, work with local businesses and relevant sites to get your Web address listed. By increasing the number of relevant incoming links, you will increase your search engine ranking and improve the popularity of your site. Basically, find areas where your patients and potential clients will benefit from finding your Web address. Try to make your site as accessible as possible.

Check the search engines

Make sure your site is available via search engines. Try various searches on engines such as *yahoo.com*, *msn.com*, *google.com*. If you aren't listed, ask your Web design team to explain and address.

Keep it up to date

Make sure the information on your Web site stays relevant and current. Make sure all dates on the site get revised as time changes. If you have a news section, make sure news is posted frequently. If a visitor comes to the site and sees the last update was 2 years ago, that may affect his impression of your practice.

If you have phone numbers and e-mail addresses on the Web site, make sure someone is available on the other end. If patients and potential clients e-mail your practice with no response, that's bad customer service. Your Web site should never take the place of quality customer service. It's an extension of your front office and should be treated as a competent employee.

Make sure your Web site continues to represent your brand. If your logo or marketing materials change, update the Web site. If your staff or doctors change, reflect those changes on the Web site. The Web site should be the easiest piece of marketing material to update and will have the greatest reach of all your materials of communication.

Continue testing

Try your Web site on multiple platforms (Mac, Windows operating systems) and Web browsers (Internet Explorer, Firefox, Safari). Your site should look the same everywhere and for all visitors.

Monitor the progress

Review traffic data from time to time. See how many people visit, where they come from, and what pages they visit. These data can be provided by tools such as Google Analytics, Stat Monitor, and other free services. Ask your Web design firm to set up this service for your Web site. A script will need to be added to your Web site. You will be able to access these reports online at any time.

In addition to traffic reports, solicit feedback from your patients regarding the site. Have they seen it? Is the information helpful? Did they print out patient forms before their visit? What did they like? What didn't they like? This can be a casual conversation during a consultation or procedure.

Evolve site content

Last but not least, continue to evolve your Web site. Browse other sites, get ideas for future enhancements, and add features. Develop ideas for what might benefit your audience and find ways to evolve the site. It's a marketing medium that lends itself to continuous change. The internet is a living medium, and your Web site can grow along with your practice.

Ask the front desk staff what typical questions they receive from patients. Can that information be added to a frequently asked questions page on your Web site? Is that information on your site now but not easy to find? Can some of this information be added to the homepage in plain view? Find ways that you can improve your customer service and reduce front desk burden by using your Web site. This is a great way to improve efficiency, employee morale, and patient relations.

Additional Readings

Dental practice websites: creating a Web presence. Dent Clin North Am 2002;46(3):463–75 PMID: 12222091 http://tinyurl.com/27k427.

Hire the Internet to manage your practice. Tex Dent J 2002;119(4):366–8 PMID: 11977900. http://tinyurl.com/28utcp.

Does your practice website need updating? Br Dent J 2005;198(5):259–60 PMID: 15870742. http://tinyurl.com/2dbppu.

Advanced marketing strategies to build the esthetic dental practice. Alpha Omegan 1994;87(4):13–6 PMID: 9470523. http://tinyurl.com/2buc3g.

Ten top tips: building a great dental website. Tex Dent J 2005;122(5):484–6 PMID: 16022486. http://tinyurl.com/yqbkks.

Developing a value-added Web site. Healthc Financ Manage 2000 Mar;54(3):40–6 PMID: 10847914. http://tinyurl.com/22kwsm.

References

[1] Creating a practice website. Br Dent J 2007;202(10): 597–604 PMID: 17534318 Available at: http://tinyurl.com/ytnpq2.

[2] Branding your practice: twelve practical steps to creating lifelong patient relationships. J Med Pract Manage 2005;20(5):266–70 PMID: 15921141. Available at: http://tinyurl.com/22kuyj.

[3] Practical marketing for dentistry, 8. Communication strategies, identifying audiences and developing messages. Br Dent J 1996;181(5):180–5 PMID: 8854427. Available at: http://tinyurl.com/2x6m48.

[4] Effective website promotion. Alpha Omegan 2006; 99(3):126–7 No abstract available. PMID: 17216763. Available at: http://tinyurl.com/38e3dy.

[5] Current price trends from Godaddy.com, Networksolutions.com and Register.com.

The Successful Oral and Maxillofacial Surgery Practice

Colin S. Bell, DDS, MSD[a,b,*]

[a]Department of Oral and Maxillofacial Surgery, Baylor College of Dentistry,
Texas A&M University System, 3302 Gaston Avenue, Dallas, TX 75246, USA
[b]Oral Surgery Associates of North Texas, 4015 Worth Street, Dallas, TX 75246, USA

As recently as 15 years ago, it was commonplace for young oral and maxillofacial surgeons graduating from training programs and for those leaving active military service to have little difficulty establishing extremely financially successful oral and maxillofacial surgery practices. Traditional indemnity insurance typically paid well for oral and maxillofacial surgery services, and patients often had minimal out-of-pocket expense.

Today that success is no longer assured without an aggressive financial, marketing, and practice-management strategy. A number of factors are responsible for this situation, including but not limited to the following:

1. Increased market penetration of managed care insurance plans, increasingly requiring patients to have much higher copayments, deductibles, and out-of-pocket expense
2. Expanded levels of services provided by general dental practitioners that have encroached on procedures traditionally done in the offices of oral and maxillofacial surgeons
3. Changing referral patterns and boundary shifts between the traditional specialties in dentistry (ie, dentoalveolar and implant surgery being performed by periodontists and other dental specialists)
4. Ongoing and continued increases in overhead costs resulting from compliance (ie, with Health Insurance Portability and Accountability Act and Occupational Safety and Health Administration regulations) and benefits issues, primarily health care insurance
5. Increasing trends of itinerant oral and maxillofacial surgeons and dentists not trained in oral and maxillofacial surgery to provide surgical services in the general dental practitioner's office
6. Increasing levels of competition for disposable-income dollars by patients who ultimately are the consumers of oral and maxillofacial surgery

All these issues have led to an environment in which it is increasingly more difficult for practices to be successful and to maintain levels of success once they have been achieved. In the future it will be ever more important to rely on aggressive and consistent marketing strategies and on the implementation of seamless and efficient business systems to allow for continued success. Only practices that implement these methods will be able to operate in an acceptably profitable and stress-free environment.

Practice decisions

The decision-making process for young oral and maxillofacial surgeons graduating from training programs and for those exiting from active military careers typically revolves around where to practice and whether to practice solo or in a group setting. These decisions generally have to be made 6 to 12 months in advance to secure office space, coordinate construction, purchase equipment, and assemble a staff to allow timely and efficient practice inception. Compliance issues with regard to building codes have made this process more lengthy and complex.

* Department of Oral and Maxillofacial Surgery, Baylor College of Dentistry, Texas A&M University System, 3302 Gaston Avenue, Dallas, TX 75246.
E-mail address: csbell@aol.com

Practice characteristics clearly seem to be heading in the direction of group practices because of the cost efficiency and the ability to participate in a variety of different insurance networks. Although many mature practices seem to be gravitating away from managed care insurance contracts, the young oral and maxillofacial surgeons, anxious to carry out the full scope of training, will have little opportunity to carry out these procedures in most areas of the country unless they participate fully in the most widely used managed care groups in their particular geographic area. Often the credentialing process and acceptance into programs are rather lengthy, but they tend to be shortened greatly in a group practice that already participates in such plans. Generational differences for young oral and maxillofacial surgeons today, who want to be able to share call and enjoy time off, also favor group practices. Finally, a group practice offers a ready-made business model system to allow new practitioners to start actually doing oral and maxillofacial surgery procedures quickly after graduation instead of spending an inordinate amount of time on management and practice development in a new solo practice. Ideally, a group practice should have age spacing of oral and maxillofacial surgeons to reach out to and relate better to all age groups of potential referral sources.

Within group practices, there is a significant trend toward operating as an incorporated structure as a C or subchapter-S corporation, because of simplicity and the business advantages. Use of an incorporated entity generally is an efficient way to do business. This structure allows oral and maxillofacial surgeons and their employees to be paid salaries with regular and timely deductions for Social Security, Medicare, and federal income tax, making it possible to avoid miscalculations of large estimated quarterly taxes. Without appropriate planning, the oral and maxillofacial surgeon could face a large tax bill the following year, when income tax returns are due. Use of an outside or online payroll service to withdraw and pay these taxes automatically and to file all appropriate quarterly and unemployment forms on a timely basis is a great step toward simplifying the business aspect of the practice.

Markets: the patient as consumer

Oral and maxillofacial surgeons typically enter practice full of enthusiasm and bring with them a full array of surgical skills developed over many years of training. Unfortunately, most have not realized that the business of oral and maxillofacial surgery is essentially about sales. In any sales market there is a consumer; in an oral and maxillofacial surgery practice the consumer is the patient. The patient continuously deliberates whether to purchase oral and maxillofacial surgery services, which in most cases are discretionary, rather than those offered by other service sectors of the economy. For example, oral and maxillofacial surgeons compete against car manufacturers, furniture sales outlets, and other venues for disposable dollars that could be used for purchase of oral and maxillofacial surgery services. Because insurance trends clearly are beginning to place more of the financial burden on patients, recognizing that patients have the role of consumer will become even more important for financial success. In the future a successful practice will have to provide and facilitate payment methods to help patients afford oral and maxillofacial surgery services.

Equally important and surprising to the young oral and maxillofacial surgeon is the understanding of what is really important from a patient's perspective in evaluating a practice and potential quality. Most would assume the evaluation revolves solely around the personality and skills associated with the oral and maxillofacial surgeon. Initially, however, the patient's perception of a practice is determined almost solely by the first telephone contact and staff interaction at the front desk. Because, unlike a general dental practice, oral and maxillofacial surgery is a specialty that constantly requires new patients, this first contact is essential for flow of patients into the practice. Assuming that the initial contact is successful, and the patient actually presents for an initial encounter or evaluation, the appearance of the facility is next in order of importance. Third, the quality of printed materials follows closely behind the appearance of the office appearance. Unfortunately, the last, although not the least, consideration is the oral and maxillofacial surgeon. In most situations patients have no way of assessing the quality of care that is going to be delivered and initially make the assumption that they will be provided with competent and quality care based largely on the factors previously discussed.

Office policy manual

Perhaps the cornerstone of any successful practice, especially as it relates to dealing with employees, is the development and constant review of a written office policy manual. This manual initially should include a mission statement, which need not be lengthy but will help to convey to patients and employees the view of the practice from the eyes of the oral and maxillofacial surgeon. It should give employees some insight as to the philosophy of the oral and maxillofacial surgeon in practice and shed some light on the future direction of the practice. This manual should contain concise job descriptions for all employee positions, which need to be made available in advance for use in adding new staff. These job descriptions should be reviewed annually and revised as needed. They should be descriptive enough to allow new employees to read the manual and have a reasonable understanding of the responsibilities delegated to them. Specific hours of operation as well as policies regarding absences and time off should be detailed appropriately. Explanations of fringe benefits available, including health care, retirement plans, and other benefits, should be outlined in a summarized fashion to allow ease of understanding.

Policies for dealing with emergency situations and exact procedures for scheduling for maximum efficiency should be included. Oral and maxillofacial surgeons should always remain aware that emergencies often represent problems within the general dental office, an office that is the lifeblood of referrals for most oral and maxillofacial surgeons. These emergencies often do not require urgent treatment but do require an encounter to evaluate the patient to help solve the problem for the general dental practitioner.

A copy of the office policy manual should be given to each employee upon joining the practice, and each employee should be expected to give a signed statement that they have received the manual and have read it and understand all of its contents. This process eliminates future potential misunderstandings about policies and guidelines, especially in the event of employee dismissal and potential wrongful dismissal litigation.

Additionally, detailed information with regard to scripting should be included in the policy manual. Scripting is simply having set conversations to deal with the most common and even uncommon situations that are dealt with on a day-to-day basis in an oral and maxillofacial surgery practice. This information eliminates confusion and also gives great guidance to a new employee on exactly how to handle specific situations. Scripting for new-patient encounters at the front desk, financial matters, scheduling, and emergencies can help make the practice more streamlined, efficient, and profitable. If an employee is confused about how to deal with a patient encounter, the potential patient is likely to be confused also and is less likely to follow through with treatment.

Staffing

In oral and maxillofacial surgery practice, staffing levels can vary tremendously from to practice, but as a general rule approximately four full-time employees per oral and maxillofacial surgeon are the minimum for an effective and efficient practice. Specific guidelines for training individuals and those responsible for training should be included in the office policy manual. Every effort should be made to retain key and productive employees because it is estimated that the cost of training a new employee often can be close to $10,000 to 15,000. Additionally, the stress associated with the inefficiencies of losing the key employee and training a new one cannot be calculated on a dollar basis. Compensation issues should be detailed to employees in a total-compensation sheet that outlines salary and additional benefits, including health insurance, retirement plan benefits, unemployment taxes, and matching Social Security and Medicare taxes that are paid on behalf of each employee by the practice; these issues should be outlined at least on an annual basis. It is naive today to assume that from an employee's perspective compensation revolves solely around salary. Of equal importance is the feeling of great value and contribution to the practice as well as time off from routine office activities.

An office manager for a solo practice or an administrator for a group practice is essential for efficient operation. This individual should have the sole responsibility for employee evaluations, additions, and dismissals. The oral and maxillofacial surgeon operates most efficiently doing surgery and dealing minimally with other nonsurgical issues.

Although much of the ongoing daily management of an oral and maxillofacial surgery practice can be delegated to an office manager or administrator, certain duties cannot be delegated beyond the oral and maxillofacial surgeon or the managing oral and maxillofacial surgeon in a large group practice. Coordination between the certified public accountant and the oral and maxillofacial surgeon can help develop simple business systems to help crosscheck day sheets, bank receipts, and audit trails to minimize the risk of embezzlement in practice. Likewise parameters can be identified to track quickly the progress and to measure the efficiency of the business systems implemented. No single individual in the practice can be given sole responsibility for managing all financial matters in the practice.

Overhead expense

One of the key barometers of the health of an oral and maxillofacial surgery practice is overhead expense. Typically the overhead expense should range from 45% to 50% of net collections, with all revenues other than overhead expenses being designated as profit. Profit includes compensation to the oral and maxillofacial surgeon as well as all qualified plan contributions and other fringe benefits that are taken in lieu of salary. Facility charges or rent typically should range between 5% and 7% of net collections (net collections being gross collections minus refunds to patients and third-party carriers). If the oral and maxillofacial surgeon or group owns the office building or facility, the rent charge should be the highest possible in the prevailing area to provide an additional income stream to the oral and maxillofacial surgeon. Typically this can be done through a building corporation or a limited liability company that often can be used to shift high-income dollars from the oral and maxillofacial surgeon to children for future educational expenses. Staff salaries and compensation should range between 18% and 23% of annual net collections.

Supplies, including both medical and dental supplies, should range between 7% and 9%. The medical supply charge for oral and maxillofacial surgery practices performing large numbers of implant procedures could be significantly greater because of the expense involved in the purchase of implant fixtures and supplies. Other expenses include utilities, legal and accounting, dues, continuing education, and payroll taxes, including Social Security (6.2%) and Medicare (1.45%), as well as federal and state unemployment and workmen's' compensation insurance.

Additionally, insurance costs, including health, professional liability, and property and casualty coverage, must be included in overhead costs, and this particular category continues to grow steadily. In health insurance coverage, future trends will lean toward greater utilization of health savings accounts, which provide an Individual Retirement Account–like savings account that can be carried forward from one year to the next in addition to a very high-deductible health insurance policy. Trends away from traditional indemnity or Preferred Provider Organization/Health Maintenance Organization health insurance contracts toward health savings accounts will become much more prevalent in years to come. This development will, however, place a greater burden on the individual employee and patient for an increasing share of health care costs.

The cost of postage is also a category that should be strongly considered. Typically the use of a postage meter is the most effective way of minimizing postage costs. The meter should be placed in the front office to discourage personal use. Likewise exact weight can be obtained to minimize overuse of postage when one simply guesses at the weight of the particular package.

Finally, professional development and marketing should range from a minimum of 2% to a maximum of 5% of net collections. In today's competitive environment this expense should be regarded as an investment and as an acquisition cost for new patients, who are unquestionably the most important commodity in the growth of a successful practice management. Marketing is discussed in greater detail later in this article.

Allied relationships

Several important allied and professional relationships are critical to success in an oral and maxillofacial surgery or in any health care practice. An attorney with experience and health care issues is essential for the review of leases and other entities of organization, such as corporations, limited liability companies, partner/shareholder agreements, and transactions.

A certified public accountant knowledgeable in health care and dentistry likewise is paramount to financial success. The certified public accountant should be used to provide sound business and tax planning advice. Routine functions, such as quarterly payroll reports and filing of unemployment insurance tax forms, can be outsourced to an electronic payroll service, however.

All practices at one time or another need effective banking relationships. The most effective and streamlined relationships deal with private banking departments in banks that have the ability to be flexible and meet the needs of the oral and maxillofacial surgery practice. Additional relationships include those associated with certified financial planners, insurance brokers, and retirement plan specialists who are necessary to plan, implement, and carry out successful oral and maxillofacial surgery practice-management and retirement strategies.

Again, the oral and maxillofacial surgeon is most effective in providing oral and maxillofacial surgery and providing quality care for patients. Use of selected and knowledgeable consultants will help organize the practice business structure, streamline business systems, and maximize profits.

Fee schedule

Next to acquiring patients, perhaps the next most important aspect in the financially successful practice is the development of a well-considered, comprehensive, and calibrated fee schedule. For any particular geographic location, insurance database information based on zip codes is readily available for purchase. Most of this information is broken down by percentile practice for each medical and dental procedure code. Ideally, this database should be used at the inception of a practice to construct a comprehensive fee schedule for all procedural codes anticipated by the practice. For simplicity, in January of each calendar year fees should be raised across the board by a consistent percentage based on variety of different factors, primarily the cost of living, the rate of inflation, and increased cost of supplies. Employee raises and salary adjustments should be made at the same time and only at this time. Grouping these two events together provides a better sense of practice budgeting and assists office personnel in being full, equal, and supporting partners in presenting these fee increases to patients in treatment planning during the upcoming year. Employees quickly recognize that without fee increases, there could be no increases in employee salaries, compensation, or bonus packages. The database should be revisited approximately every 3 years to make across-the-board adjustments based on the procedure mix currently being performed.

Financial policy

After setting an appropriate fee schedule, each office must develop a financial policy that very specifically details how financial encounters with patients should be performed. This policy should include methods to evaluate current insurance coverage and to provide patients with alternatives to cover out-of-pocket costs. This policy must be in writing and must be specific enough to deal with all contingencies. In virtually every circumstance it is more efficient and less stressful for the office staff to deal with these financial issues and fee discussions with patients rather than having the oral and maxillofacial surgeon become involved. Efficient collection policies should allow no more than 1% to 1.5% of uncollectible debt.

Additionally, because many oral and maxillofacial practices are tending toward fee-for-service and noninsured procedures, such as implant and ancillary implant services, it is imperative for oral and maxillofacial surgery practices to offer some type of alternative third-party financing. In the current economic climate, in which consumers can buy cars, houses, and furniture for no money down and extended payments, oral and maxillofacial surgeons increasingly find themselves in a competitive environment for disposable dollars, and their share seems to be shrinking with each passing year. Nevertheless, guidelines in each office should be established for the minimal amount to be considered for third-party financing. Generally it is not efficient to use third-party financing for amounts less than $1000. From a consumer standpoint, the most important aspects of alternative financing include, in descending order:

1. Down payment (The down payment should be as low as possible, and for some patients will need to be zero. Consumers can buy high-dollar consumer electronic items and cars today for little, if any, money down.)
2. Monthly payment (The monthly payment ideally should be in the range of $150 to $200/month if possible.)
3. Payment terms, not to exceed 48 to 60 months
4. The total amount financed
5. Interest rate

Today the amount of the monthly payment coupled with the minimum down payment often determines whether a patient decides to have a fee-for-service procedure performed.

Key indicators

Although there are many good practice-management software systems providing a variety of different reports, only a very few parameters determine the health of an oral and maxillofacial surgery practice. Perhaps the key element is the growth in the number of new patients seen on an annual basis. A practice that continues to generate increasing numbers of new patients every year likewise will show increases in the number of intravenous anesthetics, implants, and other productive procedures. On a monthly basis at the very minimum, the following parameters should be evaluated:

1. Number of new patients
2. Number of intravenous anesthetics
3. Number of implants
4. Production
5. Collections
6. Adjustments

This evaluation should be done for each oral and maxillofacial surgeon in a group and for each office in a multidoctor, multioffice practice. These numbers should be evaluated with respect to comparable periods in past years. This evaluation is especially important, and the time needed generally is no more than 2 to 4 hours per week for an individual or in total doctor time in a group practice.

Additional financial parameters that must be evaluated include adjustments, generally in the form of courtesy discounts. These adjustments should be less than 2% of net collections. Accounts receivable generally can range between 1.5 and 2 months of production. This amount, of course, can depend on the volume of hospital procedures done. Less than 20% of accounts receivable should be older than 90 days.

Scheduling

No single aspect of an oral and maxillofacial surgery practice can create more chaos or more efficient operation than scheduling. Because oral and maxillofacial surgeons are trained in a large variety of surgical, diagnostic, and evaluative encounters, it is imperative to group together similar types of procedures and appointments. A schizophrenic schedule that includes a surgery followed by a postoperative visit followed by a consultation followed by an emergency often becomes chaotic, tiring, and stressful for all involved. Although no one formula works best for all practices, scheduling surgeries in the mornings and all day Friday, and reserving afternoons for minor procedures, evaluations, postoperative visits, and consultations is a good starting point for most practices.

Marketing

Marketing, which is covered more extensively in another article in this issue, is critical for practices that wish to grow each year and be successful financially. From a business standpoint, marketing represents an opportunity cost and investment in the future growth in the practice. It is a method of developing ongoing and consistent relationships with potential referring sources. These relationships revolve around communication, continuing education, and other services that are of benefit to the referring office. The referral source benefits from knowing that the patient referred for an implant case or a third molar case will be taken care of well, but the major benefit in this referral lies with the oral and maxillofacial surgeon. On the other hand, as previously discussed, dealing with an emergency is a situation that generally helps the referring doctor alleviate a potential problem in his or her day's schedule. Recognition of this relationship is paramount to developing an effective marketing strategy to assist the practice's future growth. It should be the goal of each oral and maxillofacial surgery practice to convince or persuade a potential referring source of the reasons why patients should be referred to their office rather than to that of a competitor. Effective, well-thought-out, and consistent marketing is no longer an option but is an essential strategy to assure future growth.

Especially in a multidoctor practice, it is wise and efficient to delegate all marketing efforts to one employee, preferably a full-time employee, to carry these efforts out consistently and to schedule all meetings and marketing events with consistent reporting back to the oral and maxillofacial surgeon. An increasing number of practices are using full-time marketing personnel, simply because of the lack of consistency that arises when this task is performed by a variety of different employees who have other significant responsibilities for the practice. Unfortunately, a marketing strategy delegated to multiple employees often yields minimal results.

Financial independence

One of the goals for any successful health care practice, including oral and maxillofacial surgery, is a clearly defined pathway to financial independence. This goal remains elusive for a large number of health care providers, including oral and maxillofacial surgeons, who, although bright individuals, often become occupied with many other personal and practice-related issues and simply fail to plan for the future. As a result, as retirement looms closer, high debt loads accumulate, taxes are overpaid, and savings are insufficient for retirement. Early in practice a comprehensive and written financial plan should be drawn up for each oral and maxillofacial surgeon to identify the key elements and their timing to provide a direct and measurable pathway to financial independence. Such a plan can significantly reduce daily stress and increase the enjoyment in the practice.

Summary

Oral and maxillofacial surgery has been and will continue to be one of the premiere health care specialties in the United States. Incomes of oral and maxillofacial surgeons are among the highest of any profession in the country. With efficient scheduling, organized business systems, efficient fee schedules, and appropriate use of consultants, oral and maxillofacial surgery can lead to a lifestyle that is relatively stress free and that provides a great public service.

Acknowledgment

Efficient practice management in oral and maxillofacial surgery is often much more an applied art than a science. Many of the fundamental business management practices and systems necessary for success are based on years of experience, not necessarily on any particular scientific body of research or investigation. The development of the practice-management philosophy espoused in this article results in no small part from the influence of several individuals who have served as consultants for the author and his oral and maxillofacial surgery practice.

The author first acknowledges Samuel C. Rice, CPA, who has provided valuable tax planning and business advice for the past 25 years. One of the true experts in the field of practice and financial management as well as retirement planning, providing invaluable advice to the author through the years, has been John McGill, MBA, JD, CPA. Randall Johnson, JD, is a contract attorney who consistently through the years has provided simplified, timely, and efficient consultations regarding contracts, partnership agreements, partnership/buy-sell agreements, and estate planning. William H. Skelton, MBA, CFM, CRPC, has provided tremendous insight and guidance with regard to financial and retirement planning.

The Transition from Resident to Private Practice – Important Financial Decisions

Jeffrey E. Wherry, CFP®, CLU, ChFC[a],
Kenneth Thomalla, CPA, CFP®, CLU[b],*

[a]*T&H Financial Group, 3132 Wilmington Rd., New Castle, PA 16105, USA*
[b]*Treloar and Heisel, Inc., 11512 W. 183rd Street, Unit NW, Orland Park, IL 60467, USA*

Hierarchy of financial planning

Proper financial planning follows a defined structure: visualize the future, develop the strategies to accomplish this vision, and implement the strategies. Oral Surgeons would not perform a procedure without first conducting a comprehensive examination and diagnosis. Financial strategies, which are among life's most important decisions, also must be made through a coordinated plan based on the same analytical process. The financial pyramid concept illustrates the hierarchy of financial planning (Fig. 1). A proper base forms the foundation to support any strong structure. Financial planning follows the same formula. Start with the base and then move to the next level once the foundational steps are completed. Unfortunately, some dental specialists skip some elements of the base and move to the next level, ultimately leaving a shaky foundation.

The financial plan

Goals and objectives

A financial blueprint, the financial plan, starts with defining goals and objectives. These important questions should be answered:

- What is important about money to me (eg, security, freedom, power)?
- How am I controlled by money (saver, spender)?
- What needs must I address in the next couple years (eg, reinvesting in the practice, paying down debt, purchasing home)?
- What standard of living do I want to maintain?
- What are my long-term goals (eg, retirement, education)?
- What resources do I have to achieve these goals?

Analyze

Once goals are defined, the next step is to determine what steps must be taken to make these objectives a reality. Critical financial plan elements are as follows:

- Spending plan with cash flow mapping
- Insurance protection
- Debt management
- Asset allocation/investment management policy
- Target savings required for retirement, education, and other accumulation goals
- Tax management
- Asset protection
- Estate planning

Implement, monitor, and adapt

A well-written financial plan includes an action plan—a list of activities that must be undertaken to make goals a reality. Success of the plan depends on completion of the action items. No plan exists in a vacuum. Variable factors, such as practice growth, family changes, and economic conditions, all impact the overall viability of the financial plan. Plan data should be analyzed

* Corresponding author.
E-mail address: kthomalla@th-online.net (K. Thomalla).

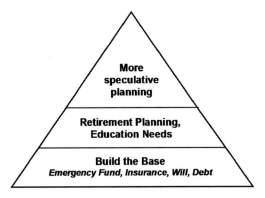

Fig. 1. The financial pyramid concept illustrates the hierarchy of financial planning.

periodically and strategies adjusted to conform to life's changes.

Build your base

The financial base covers four important areas.

Emergency fund

New practitioners should maintain a strong cash position. Set aside 3 to 6 months of living expenses in a liquid account, such as a savings account, money market, or other liquid account. This account is not an investment or spending account but rather a fund for emergency expenditures, such as insurance deductibles, major home repairs, funds to cover the waiting period on disability insurance, and other unexpected needs.

Spending plan

Success of a financial plan stems from control of spending and good savings habits. Controlling spending habits and practicing the discipline of delayed gratification are often difficult financial tasks for dental specialists. New practitioners should prepare a budget with a fixed spending limit. Spending can be adjusted upward as income increases. Consistency helps to ensure the discipline of a spending plan, so a predetermined monthly draw should be established to cover fixed spending. Often it helps to create a cash flow map—a predetermined distribution of your monthly and periodic income. For instance, each month a certain amount of dollars might be directed to:

- Monthly checking for spending purposes
- A tax account
- A college savings account
- A periodic spending account for vacations and other periodically recurring expenses

Quarterly and annual distributions might be earmarked for retirement and other accumulation accounts.

Follow wise debt rules

Generally, personal debt, not including practice acquisition loans, should not exceed 30% of gross income. This figure may be unrealistic in the first year of practice but should be adhered to in following years. Additional debt rules to observe are as follows:

- Recognize the difference between "good debt" and "bad debt." Good debt buys an appreciating asset, such as your home, or an income stream, such as your practice income. Good debt includes student loans, practice loans, and home mortgages. Bad debt purchases depreciating assets or expenditures with no residual value, often at high interest rates. Credit card and consumer debts are examples of bad debt.
- Do not accelerate debt payment if the interest rate on the loan is less than the rate of return of a moderate growth investment.

Purchase insurance

Insurance is another important pillar of your financial base. Everybody faces certain perils in life that can result in a significant financial loss. Examples of these perils are premature death, disability, catastrophic medical expenditures, property damage or theft, and professional and personal litigation. The purchase of insurance transfers the risk to the insurance company, which provides money when none exists to replace the loss from these perils. Insurance trades a potentially unaffordable loss (the cost of the peril) for a known, affordable cost (the premium). Typically, only unaffordable losses should be insured, even if the risk of occurrence is relatively low.

Create a basic estate plan

Most new practitioners do not think much about estate planning. In fact, most new practitioners do not even realize that they have an estate! Considering that many practitioners end residency with loans in excess of $200,000, it is easy to see why many believe that they do not have to plan for their estate distribution. Many of these individuals actually have items that they would like to pass to an intended recipient, however. No matter the net worth of an individual, a will is often the minimum estate planning strategy needed by all. Later in life—and beyond the scope of this article—other estate planning tools are necessary to ensure that an estate is distributed in the intended and most tax-efficient manner.

When an individual dies without a will, it is known as dying intestate. If a person dies intestate, the estate is distributed by the laws of the state in which the person resides. Often the distribution rules established by the states are not in sync with how a decedent would like to have their estate distributed. For example, most new practitioners would like to have their spouses receive their entire estate upon their death. Some intestate laws distribute these funds to the spouse and children and other family members, however. A will provides a vehicle for parents to determine who will take care of their children upon their deaths. Without a will, the courts determine the guardian for minor children. In the absence of a will, the state determines the executor, and it may not be the person the doctor desires. Initiating a will allows the doctor to choose the executor, which saves survivors significant legal footwork at an already difficult time.

Insurance policies

Depending on an oral surgeon's practice situation, associate, or owner, the following insurance plans may be required.

Disability income insurance

An oral surgeon's ability to perform their occupation is, in effect, their "production line." Inability to perform these functions because of a disability can cause great financial loss. Disability income insurance should be purchased by a new practitioner immediately upon entering practice, if not while a resident. Disability income insurance is purchased in monthly increments. Companies limit the amount of available coverage to approximately 40% to 60% of income. The amount of coverage available, as a proportion of income, decreases as income increases. Income documentation must be provided to purchase benefits, although residents often may buy a stated amount of coverage without proof of income. Several important provisions must be evaluated when purchasing disability income insurance.

Policy ownership

A "noncancelable, guaranteed renewable" policy prohibits the insurance company from increasing rates or changing policy provisions to the detriment of the policyholder. It is the recommended type of policy for dental professionals and is typically available through local agents. Many association group policies are "conditionally renewable," which allows the insurance company to increase rates and alter policy definitions. Although conditionally renewable plans often have lower rates than noncancelable, guaranteed renewable policies, a rate or definition change could leave the oral sugeon with inadequate coverage. Some professional associations endorse noncancelable, guaranteed renewable policies with a discounted premium. These plans often offer the best of both worlds: strong definitions at more affordable rates.

Definition of total disability

The best policies pay benefits when you are unable to perform the "material and substantial duties of your regular occupation." A policy with an "own occupation" definition of disability pays full benefits if you cannot perform your regular occupation (oral surgery) even if you go to work in another occupation. Rates for own occupation policies are typically the most expensive. A modified version of own occupation is one in which benefits are paid if you cannot perform your regular occupation (oral surgery) as long as you choose not to work at another occupation. Under these policies, income loss benefits actually may be paid under a partial disability policy while the insured is engaged in another occupation.

Partial/residual disability

In many cases, an oral surgeon may suffer from an illness or injury yet still work part time at his or her occupation. Partial disability, often referred to as "residual disability," pays partial benefits based on income loss when the policyholder is disabled but still working at the occupation. Some companies include residual disability in the base contract, whereas others provide it as an optional rider at an additional cost.

Elimination period

Benefits usually do not begin at the first day of disability. An elimination period, typically 90 days from the first day of disability, must be satisfied, after which time benefits commence.

Benefit period

The length of time benefits are paid during a disability is referred to as the "benefit period." Choose a benefit period that pays benefits to age 65 at a minimum. Benefit payments for life, depending on the age of disability, are available as an optional rider on some plans, whereas others might offer a rider that makes contributions to retirement plans during a disability.

Cost-of-living rider

Even at a modest 3% inflation rate, income must double over 24 years to keep pace with inflation. If a disability were to occur at a young age, benefits would have to increase to maintain purchasing power. An important optional rider, cost-of-living, increases benefits during a disability and is usually tied to changes in the consumer price index.

Additional purchase option

To buy disability insurance, a prospective insured must prove good health. Under a noncancelable, guaranteed renewable policy, the insurance company cannot later restrict or cancel the policy based on negative changes in the insured's health. The insurance company can refuse to increase coverage or increase at less-than-favorable terms, however, if the insured suffers subsequent health problems. Most companies offer optional riders that allow the insured to purchase additional coverage later, as long as income meets stated benefit issue limits, with the same terms and conditions of the existing policy, even if the insured were to experience a health problem that would otherwise render him or her uninsurable.

Life insurance

A new practitioner may need life insurance for three specific situations:

1. Personal needs: to provide income for family members.
2. Collateral for a business loan. Many banks require life insurance to be assigned as collateral for practice loans.
3. Funding for a business buyout agreement. Life insurance provides funding to purchase remaining practice value from a deceased partner's estate.

How much coverage is appropriate? In the case of loan collateral or buyout agreements, the amount of coverage is equal to the stated need of the loan or agreement. Programming coverage for personal needs is more nuanced, however. Often stated guidelines, such as "eight times income," may over- or underinflate the actual need. A basic mathematical computation provides a more accurate figure.

- Lump sum needs: amount needed to pay off debt and prefund other obligations.
- Income needs: the present value of the annual income required by the family and for how long.
- Add lump sum needs and income needs and subtract existing liquid assets.

This formula does not factor in potential social security benefits or inflation. A qualified insurance professional may use computation software for more advanced calculations. "Term" and "Permanent" are the two general classifications of available life insurance.

Term life

Term life insurance covers temporary needs and provides only pure protection without any cash accumulation. Rates start low but increase, becoming prohibitively expensive at some point in time. Multiple term life policies are available, including term with annually increasing premiums and level premium term for 10, 15, 20, and 30 years. With level rate plans, premiums increase exponentially at the end of the stated time period. A buyer should purchase the term policy with a level premium period that corresponds to how long coverage is required.

Permanent life

Permanent life insurance provides policy protection for life and cash accumulation within the policy. Premiums are set for the term of the contract, whereas the policy develops an accumulation value on a tax-deferred basis. At some point, the policy cash value may be sufficient to reduce or eliminate the premium or be drawn on as income. Permanent life is sold in several variations, including whole life, universal life, and variable life. Although significantly higher in premium than term life at the outset, permanent life costs less over a lifetime. Because of the low cost, term life likely provides the bulk of coverage throughout most of an oral surgeon's career. Permanent life also may be implemented, however, to augment retirement and estate planning strategies and provide financial flexibility later in life.

Auto insurance

Although most states require the purchase of auto liability insurance, individuals still must be aware of the risk involved with being underinsured. Most individuals insure their autos with the following coverage: liability, comprehensive, collision, and uninsured/underinsured motorists. Liability coverage insures a driver against claims made by other drivers as a result of an accident. Bodily injury, property damage, and medical payments are the three components of liability protection. Many states mandate certain limits of liability, and especially if a dental professional has a personal umbrella policy, the limits far exceed those required by their state. Individuals without a personal umbrella liability policy should ensure that their auto liability coverage is adequate. A doctor exposed to an auto liability claim risks personal assets if underinsured.

Comprehensive and collision protection insures the physical damage to the insured's auto. Comprehensive coverage insures the damage that arises from a covered peril other than collision. Uninsured/underinsured coverage protects the oral surgeon in case the other driver who was responsible for an accident lacks adequate coverage of his or her own. In this case, the doctor's coverage essentially takes the place of the driver's, who did not have adequate auto insurance. Because many new autos provide roadside assistance or similar protection, it may not be necessary to carry towing and rental coverage on an auto insurance policy.

Home owners'/rental insurance

Before discussing the different types of property coverage, it is imperative to begin with a discussion regarding the differences between property and casualty policies and life and health policies. The average consumer often thinks that as long as the premiums are paid, the policy owner is entitled to the benefits under a policy. This assumption is true in that an insurance company pays a covered claim as long as the premiums are paid. The amount to be paid depends on the concept of insurable interest, however. For property and casualty policies, you must have an insurable interest at the time of the claim. This means that if one's property coverage is listed on the policy at $200,000 but the property is only worth $150,000 at the time of the claim, the insured would only recover $150,000. This policy is in contrast to a life and health policy, such as term life insurance. If the insured dies and the policy was underwritten and issued for $200,000, upon death the beneficiary would receive $200,000 under a covered claim. This concept is important, especially when considering the number of properties that may be owned by an oral surgeon.

Home owners' coverage is property and casualty insurance for a true single family home, a condominium that one owns, or a home or apartment that is rented by the doctor. Home owners' coverage for a single-family home provides protection for the entire home and structures located on the property. The most significant difference with a condominium policy is that the policy pays benefits for the "drywall in." A master policy, purchased by the condominium association, usually covers the exterior of the building. A condominium owner must review the association coverage to ensure that the two policies mesh. Overlapping coverage may cost a little more; however, having a gap in coverage can be disastrous. Renter's coverage usually just covers the personal property owned by the renter. The building owner should have a policy covering the real property of the premises.

The insurance limits on any of these policies can be written on either a guaranteed replacement basis or replacement basis. Guaranteed replacement means that the insurance company pays a covered claim regardless of the limit on the policy. If the loss is lower than the limit, the insured receives the lesser of the two because of the concept of insurable interest. If the loss is more than the insured limit, however, then the policy holder is in a great position and would receive the larger amount. An insured often may intentionally underinsure to save premium dollars, knowing that full coverage is provided under this clause. Many insurance companies have eliminated the guaranteed replacement clause because of this situation.

Replacement value means that as long as the policy limit is equal to at least 80% of the actual home's replacement cost, the loss is paid up to the policy limit. This clause is reasonable and ensures that policy owners take responsibility to insure property for its fair value. By not requiring that 100% of the value be insured, this allows for some buffer room if reconstruction costs increase and the policy owner is not timely with increasing his or her limits. An inflation rider added to the policy helps keep policy limits escalating as building costs rise.

A typical home owners' policy has additional coverage for general liability and several secondary limits. One such limit is for items such as jewelry, artwork, and musical instruments. These limits are usually relatively low, and many items need to be "scheduled." When an item is scheduled, the entire appraised value is insurable and coverage is usually broadened. For example, most policies limit jewelry coverage to $2500 for theft or loss caused by a covered claim. A $10,000 diamond ring can be scheduled and insured for $10,000. It may even be possible to recover if the ring is lost, which is not a loss normally covered under the base policy. All valuable pieces of personal property should be scheduled to maintain appropriate coverage on the item.

Medical insurance

Purchasing medical insurance is possibly one of the toughest financial decisions because the dental specialist must determine if it is an employee benefit deductible through the office. Many factors come into this decision, including the health of the doctor, ability to attract qualified staff, and the doctor's own moral compass. If the professional chooses not to provide medical insurance to the staff, he or she might still be able to purchase coverage outside of the practice and deduct the costs, depending on his business structure.

There are primarily four types of medical insurance: health maintenance organization, preferred provider organization, traditional, and health savings account. Health maintenance organizations require the insured to stay within the network. These types of plans normally require that the insured visit the primary care provider, or gatekeeper, before visiting a specialist. A preferred provider organization eliminates the gatekeeper, which allows for greater flexibility compared with a health maintenance organization. Traditionally, preferred provider organizations stress preventive care and provide for annual check-ups. Traditional medical coverage provides for benefits after an annual deductible is met by the insured. After the deductible is paid, usual and customary expenses are fully covered subject to the policy's co-payment clause.

A health savings account is one of the new consumer-driven medical plans. Essentially, it allows the insured and/or the employer to deposit money, pre-tax, into an account while increasing the deductible under the medical insurance policy. Medical expenses—up to the deductible—can be paid from the deposit account, or the deposit account can be left to grow over the years, tax deferred. Health savings accounts are better suited to healthier professionals who will not exhaust the health savings account deposit account each year.

Personal umbrella liability insurance

Because of increased lawsuit risk, all dental professionals should consider a personal umbrella liability insurance policy. An umbrella policy sits on top of other coverage, such as auto and homeowners' insurance. The umbrella policy provides an additional layer of liability protection over these base policies. If an auto policy has a $500,000 liability limit and the umbrella policy has a limit of $2 million, then the insured has a potential limit of $2.5 million against a covered liability claim that results from an auto accident. The term "umbrella" is used because the one umbrella limit covers all of the underlying base policies. The limit of umbrella coverage is an individual consideration based on net worth and other risk factors.

Business insurance

Professional liability (malpractice) insurance

Professional liability, or malpractice insurance, is the backbone of any asset protection plan for an oral surgeon. Over the years, the premium rates have stabilized as anesthesia has become safer to administer. Although higher risk dental specialties should expect to pay considerably more than a general dentist for professional liability coverage, the rate falls well below that of most physicians. The two most common types of professional liability coverage are occurrence and claims-made insurance. Occurrence-type coverage provides for a new limit each year of practice. Essentially, one is insured for the procedure performed in a given year, regardless of when a claim may be filed. Thus, if an oral surgeon practices 30 years, an occurrence policy provides for 30 separate layers of coverage, one for each year of practice. This abundance of coverage would help protect the doctor in the case of claims that result from procedures taking place over multiple years.

Claims-made coverage was introduced as a way to lower initial premiums for the insured while limiting liability to the insurance company. Claims-made coverage provides insurance protection when a malpractice claim is made against a practitioner, regardless of when the procedure occurred. Unlike occurrence coverage, a limit for claims-made coverage moves with the insured. Throughout a 30-year practice, an oral surgeon with claims-made coverage has one limit in a given year that must provide coverage for claims due to all current and prior years of practice. Claims-made coverage is less expensive initially when compared with occurrence coverage; however, over a practitioner's career, the premium difference is relatively minor because the premiums for a claims-made policy increase over the first 5 years.

Professional liability limits vary between companies but usually start at $1 million/$3 million. The first number indicates a maximum limit for a given year per claim, whereas the second number is the total limit for all claims in a given year. Some feel that oral surgeons should purchase as much professional liability insurance as they can, whereas others look at the scope of their practice to determine the adequate amount of coverage. In either case, it is important to remember that a claim against an insured can extend past insurance to practice and personal assets.

A consent clause under professional liability insurance dictates when an insurance company can settle a claim. Pure consent means that the insured has the final approval as to when and if a claim is settled versus litigating until the end. This is the best definition available and gives the practitioner ultimate control over the claim. Many companies offer an arbitration clause. Under this clause, three people evaluate the merits of the claim to determine if it should be settled or litigated. The last type of consent is a silent consent clause. Sometimes referred to as a "hammer clause," consent of this type is held only by the insurance company. The insured really has no say in the settlement of a claim under a silent consent clause.

Office overhead insurance

Personal disability insurance pays benefits for the loss of personal income because of an injury or sickness. Office overhead insurance coverage insures the fixed overhead of an office. Examples of some of the covered fixed expenses include rent, staff salaries, utilities, phone, professional fees, and employment taxes. Office overhead coverage is needed by individual and group practices. Although disability and office overhead coverages are similar, some differences should be discussed. First, the elimination period for an office overhead policy should be shorter than that of a disability policy. Most planners recommend a 30-day elimination period to ensure that the fixed office expenses are covered without needing to use business or personal savings. Second, the benefit period for an office overhead policy should match the need. Because office overhead coverage is a reimbursement-type policy, expenses are only reimbursed if the expenses are the responsibility of the disabled business owner. If a buy-sell agreement calls for the disabled partner to sell shares after 12 months of a disability, it would not benefit him or her to have a 24-month benefit period on the office overhead plan. The additional 12 months of benefits, after the sale, would never be realized by the disabled practitioner.

Taxation of benefits is another difference between office overhead and personal disability insurance. Office overhead insurance benefits are generally nontaxable to the practice, although the premiums are deductible by the practice, which is in contrast to a personal disability plan. If practice is structured under a regular "C" corporation and elects to set up a qualified sick pay plan, then personal disability premiums can be deducted as a business expense. Deducting personal disability premiums causes benefit paid under this policy to becomes taxable, however. It is usually not recommended to pay personal disability premiums with pre-tax dollars because of the significant taxable event at the time of a claim.

The option to increase an office overhead policy is similar to those contained within a personal disability policy and always should be added to the coverage. This option allows increases without completing any additional medical underwriting and provides for increased flexibility in future years.

Business owner's policy, workers' compensation, and employment practices liability insurance

A business owner's policy (BOP) is a property- and casualty-type policy that contains numerous benefits. It is important to know what is covered under a BOP in relation to the contents coverage. Items such as equipment, furnishings, and other personal business property are easily determinable as contents. The insured value of real property, or property that is affixed to the space, is not always easily determined because of the previously discussed concept of insurable interest. A BOP only insures expenses when an insurable interest exists at the time of a claim. Often an office lease is not clear about—or the practitioner does not understand—who is responsible for the build-out of an office. Although sometimes it is the responsibility of the tenant (the practice), more often the build-out is the responsibility of the landlord. A lease must be written clearly and reviewed by the landlord and the practice to ensure that both parties clearly understand who is responsible for the office build-out and that their respective BOP policies contain the required content limit to provide adequate protection against loss.

Many oral surgeons own the building in which their practice is located, so it is important to keep an "at-arms-length" lease between the parties. Having a contractually clear and strong lease may help avoid complications at claim time. In addition to the content coverage, a BOP has a wide array of other coverage to protect the practitioner against loss. General liability, dental waste disposal, employee theft, and accounts receivable are a few examples of the additional coverage found in a BOP.

Workers' compensation coverage protects the oral surgery practice against claims that arise out of employment-related sickness and injury. Most states mandate workers' compensation that covers medical and disability payments for an employee. An owner/officer of a practice usually has a choice regarding whether to be covered under the office's workers' compensation policy. It is imperative to be sure that if one decides to opt out of workers' compensation coverage, medical insurance does not exclude claims covered under workers' compensation law. A significant gap in coverage could occur if the practitioner is not covered under medical and workers' compensation insurance.

Because the risk of employment-related lawsuits continues be a risk to all practices, employment practices liability insurance may help lessen the concern. This type of policy guards an employer against employment lawsuits related to hiring, firing, and sexual harassment claims. Coverage can be in the form of either defense cost or indemnity payments. Occasionally, this coverage can be purchased as a rider to a BOP; however, higher limits may not be available as a rider. A stand-alone employment practices liability insurance policy provides for higher limits and the richest contractual features.

Disability and life insurance buyout insurance

Any association of two or more practitioners should have an agreement to transfer shares of a practice upon the death or disability of one of the partners/shareholders. Regardless of the practice structure (eg, C-corporation, S-corporation, LLC, LLP), most buyout agreements are structured as either a cross-purchase or entity purchase. A cross-purchase buyout agreement states that if one partner becomes disabled or dies, the other partners have first right to buy that partner's share of the practice. Under a cross-purchase agreement, it is assumed that the entity is not involved in the sale transaction. There are tax benefits related to alternative minimum tax and subsequent sales related to a cross-purchase. In practices with more than two owners, however, a cross-purchase agreement may be cumbersome when funding with insurance because of the multiple insurance policies needed to insure all of the partners.

Under an entity buyout agreement, the entity itself buys the shares from a disabled partner or his or her estate. Essentially, the shares are redeemed and retired by the practice, and the other partners' percentage of ownership increases because of the reduction of total outstanding shares. An entity buyout agreement is beneficial when there are two or more partners in a practice. If insurance is purchased to fund an entity buyout agreement, the practice is the owner and beneficiary of each of the policies insuring the partners. A buyout agreement usually contains a clause for death and disability.

The death provision is best funded with term life insurance. The length of the term guarantee should coincide with the length of time the respective partner plans to practice. For example, a 30-year-old professional who plans to practice for an additional 30 years should purchase a 30-year level term plan. Many practices choose not to fund the disability portion of a buyout agreement. Some practices feel that if a partner becomes disabled, a newly hired associate will pay off the disabled partner. This thinking may seem logical in some areas, but care should be taken because of

> **Box 1. New practitioner financial checklist**
>
> *Cash flow and liquidity*
> - Emergency fund (3–6 months' living expenses)
>
> *Debt management*
> - Debt limited to 30% of income
> - Payoff credit cards and higher interest consumer loans
> - Review interest rates
>
> *Personal insurance*
> - Disability income insurance
>   Noncancelable, guaranteed renewable
>   Total disability
>   Residual disability
>   To age 65 or lifetime benefits
>   COLA
>   Additional purchase option
> - Life insurance
>   Personal needs, determined by formula
>   Collateral for loans
>   Buyout policies
> - Health insurance
> - Homeowner's insurance
>   Maximize liability limits
>   Insure 80% of replacement cost
>   Scheduled riders for jewelry, art, antiques, musical instruments, collections
>   Coverage correlated with property if renting or condominium?
> - Auto insurance
>   Maximize liability limits
> - Umbrella liability policy
>
> *Business insurance*
> - Professional liability
> - BOP
>   Maximize liability limits
>   Coverage limits correlated with property if renting or condominium?
> - Office overhead insurance
> - Commercial auto
> - Workers' compensation
> - Employment practice liability
> - Life and disability buyout
>
> *Estate planning*
> - Will
> - Check beneficiary designations on insurance policies and retirement plans
>
> *Spending plan*
> - Budget
> - Establish systematic savings
> - Plan for major expenses
>
> *Financial plan*
> - Target date to begin formal financial planning

the lack of certainty that a practice will find a suitable replacement doctor. A disability buyout insurance policy helps fund the disability provision and provide peace of mind for all of the partners that the disabled partner will receive the agreed-upon price at the time of the buyout. The going concern risk is eliminated when a buyout agreement is funded with life and disability insurance.

Transitioning to wealth accumulation planning

Next stage: avoid the "cash traps"

The transition from base building to wealth accumulation typically starts by the end of a practitioner's first full year in practice. Although the principles of wealth accumulation are beyond the scope of this article, young professionals should be aware of potential "cash traps" at this career point. Starting investment and tax-advantaged accumulations plans is certainly important; however, building a cash position in the first year of practice, in addition to the emergency fund, is more important to meet several common liquidity needs.

The tax cash trap

Residents typically graduate in mid-year, so earnings—and as a result taxes—are low at year end. Income by the end of the first full year is often significantly higher (sometimes up to quadruple) than the transition year, however, which results in exponentially higher taxes. Unfortunately, many practitioners do not increase quarterly tax payments commensurate with the growing tax burden and find themselves with a large tax bill due at year's end.

The home cash trap

Most new practitioners buy a home shortly after starting practice, which requires cash for such items as a down payment, moving expenses, and furnishings. A strong cash position helps to reduce the overall debt required for this purchase.

Laying the proper financial foundation by creating a realistic spending plan, managing debt wisely, purchasing the proper insurance, and instituting a basic estate plan is critical to help ensure long-term financial success. Upon completing these tasks, new practitioners are ready to begin turning the tremendous income stream created by their profession into tangible future wealth Box 1.

ORAL AND
MAXILLOFACIAL
SURGERY CLINICS
of North America

Risk Management in Oral and Maxillofacial Surgery
Steven M. Holmes, DDS[a,b,*], Debra K. Udey[a]

[a]Risk Management, OMS National Insurance Company, 6133 N. River Road, Suite 650, Rosemont, IL 60018-5173, USA
[b]South Florida OMS, 7600 Red Road, Suite 101, Miami, FL 33143, USA

Risk management: an overview

Risk management in medical and dental practice begins with the Golden Rule. Treat patients the way you would want to be treated or the way you would want your spouse, parents, or children treated. We all want to receive the highest quality of actual care in medicine and dentistry. We want the physicians and dentists who are our caregivers to listen to our symptoms and concerns, evaluate us appropriately through a complete examination and appropriate diagnostic tests, obtain outside consultation when appropriate, consider treatment options, and then discuss those options with us objectively so that we can choose our course of treatment. We want to understand the risks, benefits, and possible complications of our treatment options, including no treatment. We want the process to be legibly documented in our medical and dental records so that it can be reviewed to possibly help with additional challenges that we might face. The concept certainly sounds good and seems to be attainable.

OMS National Insurance Company (OMSNIC) insures approximately 83% of the practicing oral and maxillofacial surgeons in the United States. OMSNIC's statistics show that 15% to 17% of oral and maxillofacial surgeons are involved with at least one claim every year. Every 7 years, practicing oral and maxillofacial surgeons can expect to have one of their patients make a written request for compensation or actually file a lawsuit for an injury or a perceived injury caused by the oral and maxillofacial surgeon.

The good news is that the frequency of claims has drifted downward over the past few years; the bad news is that the severity of verdict awards and settlements is continuing to escalate. Million-dollar verdicts are commonplace, which has the effect of elevating the amounts paid in settlements. By far, the most common claims are related to procedures performed in the oral and maxillofacial surgeon's office on a daily basis, including extractions, removal of impacted teeth, placement of dental implants, and biopsies. Of OMSNIC's 6346 closed claims through 2005, 78% stemmed from these "routine" procedures. The costs of defense and indemnity payments of these claims made up 68% of the money paid out through 2005. More than $9 million has been paid in wrong tooth extraction claims alone.

Many of the factors involved in a patient bringing a lawsuit against an oral and maxillofacial surgeon are under the control of the surgeon. Modifying behavior and establishing office systems to protect against a claim are the primary tools available to reduce the risks of a lawsuit. The records of physicians and dentists are one of the biggest problems in defense of claims. Surgeons seem to be more interested in treating the next patient than taking the time to clearly document the current patient's chart. Millions of dollars are needlessly paid on defensible claims that need to be settled or are lost in court because of inadequate records.

A second major problem leading to claims and lawsuits is the lack of rapport. Not infrequently, patients begin legal proceedings against their health care providers because their doctor did not take the time to give them a reasonable

* Corresponding author.
E-mail address: sholmes@southfloridaoms.com (S.M. Holmes).

explanation or any information about their situation and their perceived injury. Plaintiffs' attorneys can supply them with a simple explanation using understandable medical and dental science, leading patients to believe that the doctor treated them in a negligent manner. Too late, a doctor comes to the conclusion that a few more minutes spent with a patient answering questions honestly and compassionately could have prevented a claim, but the opportunity was lost. Taking risk management issues seriously can make an oral surgeon's practice life easier. Unfortunately, many do not take the simple necessary steps to help limit the chances of litigation until after experiencing an emotionally painful, time-consuming lawsuit.

Background information on claims and lawsuits

State legislatures develop laws—medical and dental practice acts—that define how physicians and dentists may practice. They also make the laws governing how patients may bring lawsuits against doctors. State Departments of Public Regulation and State Boards of Dentistry and Medicine promulgate rules and regulations that further dictate and control how doctors must practice. Malpractice claims are usually filed under state tort systems. These claims are civil actions that allow a patient with an alleged injury to seek monetary damages from the caregiver who allegedly caused the injury. Malpractice is defined as the failure to meet the duty of care and/or a breach of accepted standards of care as established by the profession. Lawsuits allege that the failure or breach resulted in injury and damages to the patient.

The patient is labeled the plaintiff and the doctor is labeled the defendant in the legal action. Each is usually represented by an attorney. The plaintiff's attorney usually only recovers expenses and receives a financial reward if the plaintiff "wins." The plaintiff's attorney receives a contingency fee of 30% to 40% of the indemnity payment (the settlement amount or verdict amount). The defense attorney is usually paid on an hourly basis by the defendant's malpractice liability insurance carrier or, if uninsured, the defendant.

"Standards of care" are generally national and are based on the duty of the doctor to use the care and skill ordinarily used by reputable members of the profession practicing under similar circumstances. The defense and plaintiff use expert witness review to substantiate that the care received by the patient was or was not within the standard or care. In a case that goes to trial, the jury uses the expert witness testimony to decide if there was a breach of the standard of care.

Elements of a lawsuit

To "win" in a malpractice case, the plaintiff must prove what are known as the A, B, C, and Ds of litigation.

A. A doctor-patient relationship must exist between the patient and the doctor as defined by state law. The doctor must have accepted the patient as a patient of record in the practice. The plaintiff must prove that a doctor-patient relationship existed.
B. The doctor must have breached the standard of care. Expert witnesses on both sides testify as to whether the defendant has met the standard of care.
C. The patient's injury must have been caused by the defendant's breach of the standard of care; no other intervening causes or events could have contributed to the injury.
D. The patient must have suffered damages associated with the defendant's actions. If damages are proved, the plaintiff is compensated with a monetary award. The plaintiff's attorney can claim three types of damages:
   1. General damages are related to the pain and suffering caused by the injury to the patient.
   2. Special damages are the actual monetary costs the patient has paid for treatment or care of the alleged injury.
   3. Punitive damages can be assigned if the plaintiff's attorney can prove that the patient's damages were caused by deliberate actions of the defendant that were substantially below the standard of care.

The lawsuit process

Each state has statute of limitation laws that specify how long a patient has to file a lawsuit. These laws vary by state, but generally the statute is 2 or 3 years from when a reasonable patient knew or should have known about the injury. The time in which a minor can file a lawsuit often begins when the minor has reached the age of majority; however, this also varies by state. In an effort to limit frivolous lawsuits, certain states currently require that the plaintiff's attorney submit an affidavit or certificate of merit before an actual lawsuit can be filed. The affidavit or certificate is a statement by a similar specialist licensed to practice in the state who attests to the negligent care provided by the defendant physician or dentist. The first notice of a lawsuit received by the defendant doctor generally is a summons and complaint.

There is a short time period for the defendant to respond to the notification of the lawsuit once it is received. The time is usually 30 days, but it can vary by state. The doctor must contact his or her insurance company immediately upon receipt of the lawsuit. The failure to report receipt of these documents actually can jeopardize coverage. A copy of all of the patient's records must be forwarded to the insurance carrier immediately. The insurance company assigns counsel to formally respond to the lawsuit within the required time period. If this is not done within the specified period of time there are severe consequences, a default judgment is issued against the doctor, which holds him or her negligent on all counts involving the alleged injury without any opportunity to defend the action. The court decides the monetary amount of damages to compensate the plaintiff without a trial.

Once the formal complaint or a request for compensation has been received, the defendant doctor can only discuss the case with the assigned attorney and the insurance company. These are privileged communications that do not need to be shared with the plaintiff's attorney. Any other discussions are discoverable by the plaintiff's attorney. The surgeon must not discuss the claim with colleagues or they may be deposed to obtain information disclosed to them.

The beginning of a lawsuit involves both sides gathering information and evidence, which is called discovery. It takes the form of the collection of records from other physicians and dentists, written questions from each side (interrogatories) that must be answered, unsworn statements from the plaintiff and defendant, and sworn statements, which are depositions. They are taken in front of the plaintiff's attorney, defendant's attorney, and a court reporter. The expert witnesses retained by each side of the case evaluate all of the pertinent records and documents and make their assessment regarding the appropriateness of the care provided to the patient.

As the discovery process proceeds, a determination is made to defend or settle the case. In cases of clear liability or cases in which a determination is made that the case cannot be won in court, the claims handler attempts to effect a settlement. In most cases, settlements can be reached. In a small number of cases, however, plaintiffs are unwilling to settle for an amount that is reasonable, and the case must be tried to allow a jury to award a reasonable amount.

Cases that are clearly defensible are most often tried. The lawsuit process can be arduous and uncomfortable, but the claims handlers and the defense counsel do all they can to assist and support the defendant doctor. The court system is capricious at best, and it is impossible to predict whether everything outlined previously will go as planned. When the defense team (ie, attorney, claims handler, and doctor) works well together, however, there is often a good result.

Insurance

All forms of insurance involve the sharing of risk. The cost of insurance is determined by the anticipated costs of paying and defending claims. Premiums are actuarially determined on a state or regional basis. These rates vary by territory because of the differences in the costs of claims in that area. A loss ratio is determined by the actuary for a specific state or region, which is the total premium divided by the indemnity payments and the cost of providing the defense. Areas that are much more litigious have higher premiums than areas with fewer claims.

There are two types of malpractice insurance: claims-made insurance and occurrence policies. Claims-made insurance attaches the lawsuit to the year that the incident or claim was filed. Occurrence policies attach the claim into the year when the injury occurred, which can result in the claims being filed long after the event actually occurred and makes accurate pricing of an occurrence policy more difficult. When a doctor who has a claims-made policy stops practicing, there is no need for current coverage, but there is a need for tail coverage to cover any claims that are made after the doctor's retirement date.

Reducing risk

If there were fewer claims, less money would be spent on the costs of indemnity payments and the defense of claims, and the cost of liability insurance would go down. Risk managers at liability insurance companies have learned that the best way to decrease the frequency of claims is an aggressive risk management education process. The process includes face-to-face risk management seminars, on-line risk management seminars, creation of appropriate forms for the use of their insureds, and help with government-mandated issues. This process follows the age old rule: an ounce of prevention is worth a pound of cure.

Although the principles have been taught for years by risk managers, risk reduction really boils down to two major items: communication and documentation. Communication includes informed consent and is a major component of patient rapport. These two factors lead to most malpractice claims. Taking the time to keep detailed records and deal with patient nuances is just not attractive to health care providers. With the demands of the modern practice environment of managed care, less face-to-face patient time, and less reimbursement, we tend to move on to the next patient as rapidly as possible. Oral and maxillofacial surgeons choose the dental profession because of personality traits and professional desires that often do not make for wonderful record keepers and good listeners. Dentists are logical, scientific, skillful with their hands, and independent workers. Oral and maxillofacial surgeons thrive on performing surgery with precise skill. The unexciting chores of record keeping and communicating with patients at the patient's educational level are difficult for oral and maxillofacial surgeons. If doctors understand why malpractice claims are filed, avoid the common pitfalls that lead to a claim, and take action to prevent the pitfalls, however, an actual decrease in the cost of liability insurance can be attained.

Patient rapport

Teaching rapport is difficult, although its importance is undeniable. Because of the nature of oral and maxillofacial surgery practice, little time is spent with patients. A patient may be seen only for a consultation, the surgical procedure, and a postoperative follow-up visit. Several patients are seen for their consultation and surgery on the same day—frequently a busy day. Many patients are sedated or asleep for their surgery, and there is little time to develop rapport. Oral and maxillofacial surgeons are in a difficult position. They spend little time with patients and may not spend enough of it in good communication with them. It is hard for patients to have a warm and fuzzy feeling about someone they see for only a short period of time with little communication. Most lawsuits occur specifically because of a lack of or perceived lack of communication or an attitude problem with the doctor. Because patients have no way to evaluate the surgical skills or quality of an oral and maxillofacial surgeon, they evaluate the things they do understand. They evaluate how they were greeted by the receptionist over the telephone and when they came into the office. They evaluate how clean the office was, whether the staff or doctor was rushed, whether the doctor was arrogant. When a complication occurs, these are the things that patients remember and use to make their determination about the cause of the problem.

Anger is usually one of the causes in all types of lawsuits. People do not sue another person whom they like and trust. They sue someone when they are angry with that person over a perceived injury or injustice. One can do any number of things to increase rapport with patients. Several simple communication devices can easily be used. The first and most important is to sit down and talk to a patient. Look the patient in the eye instead of looking at the chart or writing the entire time. Talk to the patient on the same level, physically (sit down with the patient) and orally (use simple language and avoid the use of jargon or acronyms). When a patient speaks to you, do not interrupt him or her. Aside from steering the conversation away from something you might need to know, it is just plain rude. Do not anticipate what a patient is trying to say if he or she is not being clear. Ask the patient to rephrase the question or repeat it back to him or her so that you are both sure the right question is being answered.

One of the most crucial times for an oral and maxillofacial surgeon to be available for a patient is when a complication or untoward event occurs. Taking the time to sit down with the patient to explain exactly what happened and what the future course will be is critical. Give the patient time to digest the information, and let him or her know that if he or she has additional questions after the conversation, you will be available to answer them. An empathetic and reassuring voice can go a long way toward ensuring that the patient remains satisfied with the care.

Ensuring that patients are informed and feel that you are available to answer their questions and give them the information they need does much to keep them from becoming angry and turning to an attorney to obtain the information they should be obtaining from you.

Informed consent

Patients have the right to determine their course of treatment, including the choice of no treatment. Historically, informed consent comes from the legal principles of battery. Battery, a criminal act, is the intentional, unwanted touching of another person without consent or permission. The *Schloendorff v. Society of New York Hospitals* court decision in 1914 stated: "Every human being of adult years and sound mind has a right to determine what shall be done with his own body... and a surgeon who operates without the patient's consent commits an assault for which he is liable in damages."

When OMSNIC began as AAOMS Mutual Insurance Company in 1988, one of its first projects was to educate policy holders about the importance of informed consent for procedures. Informed consent is a process, not just a signed form. The process consists of educating the patient about all of the informed consent elements to develop realistic expectations before treatment. The process must be documented through progress notes and informed consent forms. Procedure-specific consent forms were developed to aid oral and maxillofacial surgeons in documenting the informed consent process.

Currently oral and maxillofacial surgeons are required to disclose the material risks and benefits of a proposed procedure that a reasonable person would want to understand to come to a decision about whether to undergo a procedure. This information includes any alternatives that are available to the patient, even if provided by another health care professional. Disclosure of possible complications of all of the alternative treatments is necessary for a patient to make an informed choice of treatments. Documentation in the patient's record of the informed consent discussion is imperative in the prevention of malpractice activity. Specific elements in the documentation of the informed consent process should be included in the informed consent form or progress notes:

- The specific medical necessity and diagnosis for the proposed treatment.
- The anticipated benefit of the proposed treatment.
- The nature of the proposed treatment and alternatives. What is involved with the proposed procedure and alternatives?
- The expected outcome of the proposed procedure and the outcomes from alternative treatments.
- The risks associated with no treatment.
- No guaranteed outcomes or results.
- Documentation of the patient's opportunity to ask questions.
- Offering the patient the opportunity to seek a second opinion before proceeding with treatment.

As a result of the educational process undertaken by OMSNIC, the frequency of lack of informed consent claims has dropped dramatically, resulting in a significant reduction in the premiums for liability insurance paid by oral and maxillofacial surgeons. That success is remarkable and worthwhile, but the process continues.

Documentation and legible records

Approximately one third of claims are deemed indefensible by claims handlers and defense attorneys because of a lack of appropriate chart notes. Malpractice insurance carriers are forced to settle too many defensible claims caused by poor records. Most training programs teach residents to document hospital and clinic patient records in a SOAP (subjective, objective, assessment, plan) format, including enough information so that if a different resident saw the patient on subsequent visits, the patient's diagnosis and the ongoing patient treatment plan would be known.

In training, an orthognathic operative report would describe precisely where incisions were made, how the flaps were reflected, where bone was cut, the amount of the movements in all directions, what type of fixation was used, how the flaps were reapproximated, and the type of sutures that were used. An implant and bone grafting operative report would describe the procedure in a similarly complete fashion. Even extraction cases have detailed operative reports. Unfortunately, once training is completed and surgeons are in their own practice, this habit frequently seems to disappear. Often, a patient's record is short and cryptic with little or no clinical information, which is especially true for cases that seem to be "simple" or "routine."

Legally we have the same requirements for our office notes. Another oral and maxillofacial surgeon should be able to read our office notes and describe how the patient's surgery was accomplished. Follow-up visit notes describe a patient's condition. This is true for every surgery or procedure performed in the oral and maxillofacial surgery offices. There is no better manner to document every patient visit than the SOAP format.

Dental and medical practice acts specify record-keeping standards. Any other similar physician or dentist should be able to read a patient's records and describe the following information:

- Patient complaints and symptoms
- Findings and results of a patient's examination
- Diagnostic tests and their results
- Discussion about the diagnosis and treatment options given to a patient
- Discussion about the risks and benefits
- Possible complications
- Options and the likely consequences of no treatment
- Surgical procedure
- Postoperative care

This record keeping applies to every patient visit, from the initial consultation to the last postoperative visit. If an oral and maxillofacial surgeon's records do not meet these requirements, the records are not up to legal standards. Brief and inadequately recorded chart notes allow the plaintiff's attorney to "paint" a picture of the patient's care that implies substandard treatment, equivalent to the chart notes.

SOAP charting helps prevent claims when used for all patient visits.

The subjective patient's complaints and concerns are listed. Listening to the patient, making eye contact, and noting the patient's statements help establish rapport. Noting these comments in the record allows a picture of the ongoing care to be "seen" far more clearly.

The objective findings, including positive and negative findings, are documented. The lack of swelling, redness, or drainage can be an important factor in defense of a claim. The presence of signs with objective descriptions (eg, size, length, induration, color) limits the latitude afforded the plaintiff's attorney in his or her descriptions of the alleged injury.

The oral and maxillofacial surgeon's assessment of the situation is documented. This is the most common factor omitted from charts. Understanding the thought process that led to the decision making is important. Remembering the patient and how the decisions were made after months or years is often difficult. Jury interviews show that if it is written in the record, it is likely to be the truth.

The plan for the patient's care is written down. Not only can the surgeon who treated the patient know what was planned but also a partner or subsequent treating surgeon knows the plan.

When a claim occurs and the record is lacking clinical details, defensible claims are frequently lost. It becomes a liars' contest in the court room. Add a believable patient and an arrogant doctor, and defensibility is even more difficult. A little effort in documenting the patient's condition and the thought process that led to the decisions easily can make the difference between a costly settlement and an appropriate dismissal. There are many ways to make legible, descriptive records easier to accomplish. Many suppliers make appropriately sized (8.5 × 11 in) patient charts and forms. Certainly medical and dental practice is past the time of the 5 × 8-in patient record card. Many liability insurance companies offer various forms, including informed consent documents, health history forms, anesthesia records, discharge criteria, and prescription logs, for their insureds to use. Some offices are paperless, with the entire patient record kept on the computer hard drive. No matter which way the records are kept, the legal requirements must be met. Patient records must be kept for the time period required by state law.

Several elements are crucial to proper chart documentation:

State law requires that a patient's record be legible (dictated and transcribed records are obviously the most legible).
All chart entries must be dated and initialed.
Every page must contain the patient's name.
All entries must be in chronologic order.
Any corrections or additions to the note must be made by the doctor in the correct manner, which is a new entry, dated when added and labeled as an addition to the note needing clarification.
Legal documentation of prescriptions as set forth by state dental and medial practice acts must include the following:
- The full name of the drug
- The strength

- The amount of pills/liquids dispensed
- How the drug is to be taken
- Number of refills

Any common, serious side effects discussed with the patient also should be recorded on the progress notes. The recording of prescriptions can be accomplished in several ways to satisfy the state requirements. The best way to keep prescription information in patient charts is a dedicated prescription log. Having every prescription listed in one location allows the surgeon, partner, or staff to have information about all drugs that have been prescribed for the patient available with little effort. This documentation can help prevent cases that involve drug addiction and overprescription of narcotic medications.

Record alterations are illegal. In some states, altering a patient's record is a felony. An alteration of a patient's record is a premeditated act. A claim in which there is even the slightest possibility of an altered patient chart cannot go to court. The plaintiff will win the case, and the doctor may be subject to criminal penalties. The insurance company has to settle the claim—frequently for much more than the claim is worth—to protect the oral and maxillofacial surgeon who has committed the illegal act. The doctor could be liable for criminal charges in addition to the civil malpractice case. The defense of criminal charges is not covered under malpractice liability insurance. The court could award punitive damages in a case in which a doctor alters the patient's record in an attempt to strengthen the defensibility of the claim. Punitive damages are not covered by most liability carriers. Handwriting experts can testify to the likelihood of an entry being an addition because of the difference in ink, spacing, or slant.

It seems that properly documenting a patient's record is a laborious, time-consuming effort. Risk managers attempt to educate their insureds that a few minutes spent documenting patient charts on a daily basis is a tremendous investment compared with the hours spent away from family and out of practice once involved in a lawsuit. With the proper forms and a few minutes of time, however, the quality of every patient's chart notes would improve tremendously.

Office practices and policies

It is imperative that good office practices and policies be put in place and used consistently to ensure the steady flow of information needed by the doctors, staff, and patients. Diagnostic tests are conducted in oral and maxillofacial surgeons' offices, patients are sent to other facilities for diagnostic tests and consultation, and pathology specimens are sent for diagnosis. Appropriate policies in the oral and maxillofacial surgery office must ensure that these procedures are conducted properly.

All radiographs obtained in the oral and maxillofacial surgeon's facility must be dated, read, and noted in the patient's record, including periapical, occlusal, panoramic, cephalometric, skull, sinus, and CT films. Maxillofacial CT units are becoming more commonplace in the surgeon's office. These scans may reveal areas of the head and neck that may be outside of the oral and maxillofacial surgeon's training. Reading these scans may present difficulty to the surgeon. The surgeon has the same liability for pathology that is evident on a panoramic film or a CT scan. If the oral and maxillofacial surgeon is not comfortable reading the radiographs taken in the office, an outside service should be contracted to review the radiographs and provide a written report. A patient cannot sign a waiver relieving the oral and maxillofacial surgeon of liability for pathology that was evident on a radiograph or scan but not recognized by the surgeon.

It is the oral and maxillofacial surgery office's responsibility to have office policies in place to ensure that all patient specimens are received by the laboratory and that the results are received in the office in an appropriate time period. All pathology and laboratory specimens must be logged out and the reports logged in. These reports must be reviewed, initialed, and dated by the oral and maxillofacial surgeon. These protocols also apply to hospitalized or outpatient surgical patients. A good practice is for the surgeon to also make an entry in the patient's progress notes regarding the diagnosis or findings.

If a patient fails to appear for the postoperative appointment and the pathology report is filed in the chart without notifying the patient of the results, disaster can occur. Office practices and fail-safe procedures must be in place to prevent laboratory or pathology reports from slipping through a crack in the system and documenting that recall patients are contacted. Lawsuits regarding failure to diagnose cancer are often ugly, painful, and costly cases for the patient and oral and maxillofacial surgeon.

Discharging patients from your practice

All health care providers have discretion in choosing the patients they accept for treatment with certain limitations. Doctors do not have a duty to accept all patients for care. The Americans with Disabilities Act prohibits withholding care "due to discrimination" for the individuals covered by the act. Managed care agreements may obligate a provider to provide treatment for all patients covered under the contract. Hospital emergency room commitments or the "on-call" schedule may limit a provider's ability to decline to care for a patient.

Establishing a doctor-patient relationship obligates the doctor to the duty of continuing care for the patient until the patient no longer requires care, the health care provider and the patient mutually agree that the care should be continued elsewhere, or the relationship is terminated by either the doctor or the patient. Providing ongoing care to patients who are uncooperative, refuse to follow instructions, and are generally noncompliant is a potential liability that the oral and maxillofacial surgeon does not have to accept. This type of patient can be discharged from care following the legal requirements of the state law. The reason for withdrawing from the patient's care does not need to be disclosed to the patient unless required by state law. Discussing the situation with the liability insurance company's claims handler or a local attorney is recommended so that all of the state requirements are met.

To discharge a patient from care, the surgeon must be certain that the patient's condition is stable. Once that fact has been established, the surgeon must send the patient a letter stating that he or she is withdrawing from the patient's care, giving a means to locate a new provider (usually providing the name and telephone number of the local dental society), and offering to provide continuing care or emergent care for the period of time stated in the state law. It is also a good idea to offer to make a copy of the patient's records available to the subsequent treater with a release that is appropriately signed by the patient. This letter must be sent by certified mail, return receipt requested, and by regular mail. The letter should be marked at the top have being sent by certified mail, return receipt requested, and regular mail.

Managed care contracts should be reviewed for the terms under which a patient may be discharged from care. The problems caused by the patient leading to the decision to withdraw from care must be thoroughly documented in the patient's record. Abandonment is an uncommon claim, and discharging patients from care is a serious decision. Seek the counsel of the insurance company's claims staff for situations that could possibly be termed abandonment.

Summary

Medical malpractice claims are a fact of life. Not every procedure performed by oral and maxillofacial surgeons has a perfect result, and our society is ever more unwilling to accept imperfect results. If there is not a sufficient basis of communication with patients that will see them through a complication or untoward result, patients may choose to seek redress through a claim or lawsuit. If the clinical chart is not appropriately documented, the chances of a successful defense are compromised. Using the principles outlined in this article can put oral and maxillofacial surgeons in a good position to decrease the number of potential claims and make the few that are filed against them eminently defensible.

Index

Note: Page numbers of article titles are in **boldface** type.

A

Academic careers, fellowship training and, **11–15**
    additional degrees, 14
    career goals, 13
    financial compensation, 13–14
    future growth of the specialty, 14–15

Advertising, to recruit associates, 30–31

Air Force, US, careers for oral and maxillofacial surgeons in, 23–25

Allied relationships, in the successful practice, 104–105

Army, US, careers for oral and maxillofacial surgeons in, 19–20

Associateships, in oral and maxillofacial surgery, planning a successful associateship and practice transition, **27–36**
        advertising and recruitment, 30–31
        analysis, evaluation, and considerations, 28
        phase 1 - trial or break-in, 32
        phase 2 - the buy-in, 32–34
        phase 3 - the buy-out, 34–36
        preparation, 28–30

Auto insurance, financial planning for transition from residency to private practice, 113

B

Benefits, for associates in oral and maxillofacial surgery practice, 30–31
    in contracts, 40

Branding, of he oral and maxillofacial practice, 92

Business insurance, 114–117
    business owner's. workers' compensation, and employee practice liability, 115–116
    disability and life insurance buy-out, 116–117
    office overhead, 115
    professional liability/malpractice, 114–115

Buy-in, into practice by associate surgeon, 32–34

Buy-out, of practice by associate surgeon, 34–36

Buy-outs, contractual concerns, 42–43

Buy-sell agreements, contractual concerns, 41–44

C

Career planning, fellowship training and academic careers, **11–15**
    in the military and Veterans Administration, **17–26**
    transitioning from residency to private practice, **1–9**

Claims, risk management and, 120–121

Compensation, for associates in oral and maxillofacial surgery practice, 33–34
    contracts for, 38

Computer technology, in oral and maxillofacial surgery, **79–89**
    in diagnostic imaging, 80–82
    in implantology, 82–84
    in orthognathic surgery, 84–87
    in stereolithographic modeling, 87–88

Cone beam technology, incorporation of, in modern oral and maxillofacial surgery office, 59–61

Confidentiality, in associate's contract, 41

Consent, informed, in risk management, 123

Consumers, patients as, in the successful practice, 102

Contracts, in oral and maxillofacial practice, **37–46**
    buy-sell, shareholder, and operating agreements, buy-outs, 42–43
    control issues, 43
    distributions, 43–44
    liability for practice's liabilities, 44

Contracts (*continued*)
    employment agreements, 38–41
        benefits and duties, 40
        compensation, 38
        confidentiality, 41
        consequences of termination, 39–40
        indemnification and insurance, 41
        ownership of intellectual property, 41
        restrictive covenants, 40–41
        terms and termination, 38–39
    letters of intent, 37–38
    technology agreements, 44–45

Control issues, in buying into practice, contractual concerns, 42–43

Credentialing, and privileging for the oral and maxillofacial surgeon, **47–54**
    current challenges to, 52
    preparing for, 50–51
    process for, 48–50
    qualifications, 47–48
    special circumstances, 51–52

D

Debt, student, factor in transition from residency to private practice, 3

Design, office. *See* Oce design.

Diagnostic imaging, computer technology in, 80–82

Digital operating system, in modern oral and maxillofacial surgery office, 59

Disability insurance, financial planning for transition from residency to private practice, 116–117

Discharge, of patients, from your practice, in risk management, 126

Distributions, contractual concerns, 43–44

Documentation, in risk management, 123–126

E

Employee relations, positive, marketing the oral and maxillofacial surgery practice through, **65–77**
    communication, 74–77
    competency and presentation, 69–70
    enthusiasm, joy, and energy, 72
    finding good employees, 67–69
    givers *versus* takers, 70–71
    offensive and defensive employees, 71
    self-management, 72
    superstars *versus* team players, 71–72
    termination, 72–74
    unconditional commitment, 70

Employment agreements, contracts for, 38–41
    benefits and duties, 40
    compensation, 38
    confidentiality, 41
    consequences of termination, 39–40
    indemnification and insurance, 41
    ownserhsip of intellectual property, 41
    restrictive covenants, 40–41
    terms and termination, 38–39

F

Fee schedule, in the successful practice, 105

Fellowship training, and academic careers, **11–15**

Financial planning, for transition from resident to private practice, **109–118**
    auto insurance, 113
    business insurance, 114–117
        business owner's. workers' compensation, and employee practice liability, 115–116
        disability and life insurance buy-out, 116–117
        office overhead, 115
        professional liability/malpractice, 114–115
    hierarchy of, 109–111
    home owner's/rental insurance, 113–114
    insurance policies, 111–112
    life insurance, 112–113
    medical insurance, 114
    personal liability insurance, 114
    wealth accumulation planning, 117–118

Financial policies, n the successful practice, 105

Floor plans, for modern oral and maxillofacial surgery office, 55–59

H

Health insurance, financial planning for transition from residency to private practice, 114

Home owner's insurance, financial planning for transition from residency to private practice, 113–114

I

Implantology, computer technology in, 82–83

Indemnification, in associate's contract, 41

Information technology. *See* Computer technology.

Informed consent, in risk management, 123

Insurance, financial planning for transition from residency to private practice, **109–118**
  in associate's contract, 41
  malpractice, 121

Intellectual property, in associate's contract, 41

Intent, letters of, 37–38

Internet service provider agreements, contractual concerns in practice, 44–45

L

Lawsuits, risk management and, 120–121

Letters of intent, 37–38

Liability, of associate for practice's liabilities, contractual concerns, 43–44

License agreements, for technology, contractual concerns in practice, 44–45

Life insurance, financial planning for transition from residency to private practice, 112–113

Location, factor in transition from residency to private practice, 2–3

M

Malpractice, risk management and, **119–126**

Malpractice insurance, 121
  financial planning for transition from residency to private practice, 114–115

Marketing, n the successful practice, 106
  of the oral and maxillofacial surgery practice, 63
    through positive employee relations, **65–77**
      communication, 74–77
      competency and presentation, 69–70
      enthusiasm, joy, and energy, 72
      finding good employees, 67–69
      givers *versus* takers, 70–71
      offensive and defensive employees, 71
      self-management, 72
      superstars *versus* team placers, 71–72
      termination, 72–74
      unconditional commitment, 70
  Web development for, **91–100**

Medical insurance, financial planning for transition from residency to private practice, 114

Military careers, in oral and maxillofacial surgery, **17–26**
  Department of Veterans Affairs, 17–19
  US Air Force, 23–25
  US Army, 19–20
  US Navy, 20–23

N

Navy, US, careers for oral and maxillofacial surgeons in, 20–23

O

Office design, for oral and maxillofacial surgery practice, **55–64**
  design concepts, 55
  digital operating system, 59
  floor plan, 55–59
  incorporation of cone beam technology, 59–61
  necessary personnel, 61–63
  practice marketing, 63

Office overhead insurance, financial planning for transition from residency to private practice, 115–116

Office policies, in risk management, 123–126

Office policy manual, in the successful practice, 102–103

Operating agreements, contractual concerns, 41–44

Orthognathic surgery, computer technology in, 84–87

Overhead expenses, in the successful practice, 104

P

Patients, as consumers, in the successful practice, 102
  discharge from your practice, in risk management, 126
  rapport with, in risk management, 122–123

Personal umbrella liability insurance, financial planning for transition from residency to private practice, 114

Personnel, for modern oral and maxillofacial surgery office, 61–63

Policies, office, in risk management, 123–126

Policy manual, in the successful practice, 102–103

Practice management, for oral and maxillofacial surgeons, 1–126
  a new beginning, 7–8

Practice management (*continued*)
  contractual concerns, **37–46**
    buy-sell, shareholder, and operating agreements, 41–44
    employment agreements, 38–41
    letters of intent, 37–38
    technology agreements, 44–45
  credentialing and privileging, **47–54**
  fellowship training and academic careers, **11–15**
    academic careers, 13–15
    fellowships, 11–13
  information and computer technology, **79–89**
  marketing the practice through positive employee relations, **65–77**
  military and Veterans Administration careers, **17–26**
    Department of Veterans Affairs, 17–19
    US Air Force, 23–25
    US Army, 19–20
    US Navy, 20–23
  modern oral and maxillofacial surgery office, **55–64**
    design concepts, 55
    digital operating system, 59
    floor plan, 55–59
    incorporation of cone beam technology, 59–61
    necessary personnel, 61–63
    practice marketing, 63
  planning a successful associateship and practice transition, **27–36**
    advertising and recruitment, 30–31
    analysis, evaluation, and considerations, 28
    phase 1 - trial or break-in, 32
    phase 2 - the buy-in, 32–34
    phase 3 - the buy-out, 34–36
    preparation, 28–30
  risk management, **119–126**
    claims and lawsuits, 120–121
    discharging patients from your practice, 126
    documentation and legible records, 123–125
    informed consent, 123
    insurance, 121
    office practices and policies, 125–126
    overview, 119–120
    patient rapport, 122–123
    reducing risk, 121–122
  the successful practice, **101–107**
    allied relationships, 104–105
    fee schedule, 105
    financial independence, 106–107
    financial policy, 105
    key indicators, 105–106
    marketing, 106
    office policy manual, 102–103
    overhead expense, 104
    patient as consumer, 102
    practice decisions, 101–102
    scheduling, 106
    staffing, 103–104
  transitioning from residency to private practice, **1–9**
    financial considerations for, **109–118**
    the beginning, 1–4
    the end, 6–7
    the middle, 4–6
  web development, **91–100**

Private practice, keys to success, **101–107**
  allied relationships, 104–105
  fee schedule, 105
  financial independence, 106–107
  financial policy, 105
  key indicators, 105–106
  marketing, 106
  office policy manual, 102–103
  overhead expense, 104
  patient as consumer, 102
  practice decisions, 101–102
  scheduling, 106
  staffing, 103–104
  transitioning from residency to, **1–9**

Privileging, of oral and maxillofacial surgeons. *See* Credentialing.

R

Rapport, with patients, in risk management, 122–123

Records, medical, in risk management, 123–126

Recruitment, of associates, 30–31

Rental insurance, financial planning for transition from residency to private practice, 113–114

Residency, financial planning for transition to private practice, **109–118**
  auto insurance, 113
  business insurance, 114–117
    business owner's. workers' compensation, and employee practice liability, 115–116

disability and life insurance buy-out, 116–117
office overhead, 115
professional liability/malpractice, 114–115
hierarchy of, 109–111
home owner's/rental insurance, 113–114
insurance policies, 111–112
life insurance, 112–113
medical insurance, 114
personal liability insurance, 114
wealth accumulation planning, 117–118
transitioning to private practice from, **1–9**

Restrictive covenants, for practice associates, 40–41

Risk management, for oral and maxillofacial surgeons, **119–126**
claims and lawsuits, 120–121
discharging patients from your practice, 126
documentation and legible records, 123–125
informed consent, 123
insurance, 121
office practices and policies, 125–126
overview, 119–120
patient rapport, 122–123
reducing risk, 121–122

S

Sale, of practice, buy-out by an associate, 34–36

Scheduling, in the successful practice, 106

Shareholder agreements, contractual concerns, 41–44

Staffing, in the successful practice, 103–104

Stereolithographic modeling, computer technology in, 87–88

Surgeons, oral and maxillofacial, common contractual concerns for, **37–46**
credentialling and privileging of, **47–54**

T

Technology agreements, contractual concerns in practice, 44–45

Termination, employee, contracts for associates, 38–39
consequences of, 39–40

Training, fellowship, and academic careers, **11–15**

Transitions, associateship and practice, **27–36**
from residency to private practice, **1–6**
financial planning for, **109–118**

U

United States military, careers for oral and maxillofacial surgeons in, **17–26**
Department of Veterans Affairs, 17–19
US Air Force, 23–25
US Army, 19–20
US Navy, 20–23

V

Veterans Administration, careers for oral and maxillofacial surgeons in, 17–19

W

Wealth accumulation planning, for transition from residency to private practice, 117–118

Web development, for oral and maxillofacial surgeons, **91–100**
costs of, 93–96
how to get started, 96–99
reasons for a practice Web site, 91–93
updating and maintaining your site, 99–100

Moving?

Make sure your subscription moves with you!

To notify us of your new address, find your **Clinics Account Number** (located on your mailing label above your name), and contact customer service at:

E-mail: elspcs@elsevier.com

800-654-2452 (subscribers in the U.S. & Canada)
407-345-4000 (subscribers outside of the U.S. & Canada)

Fax number: 407-363-9661

Elsevier Periodicals Customer Service
6277 Sea Harbor Drive
Orlando, FL 32887-4800

*To ensure uninterrupted delivery of your subscription, please notify us at least 4 weeks in advance of move.